BLIND—AND I SEE!

BLIND—
AND I SEE!

Robert Weller

Publishing House
St. Louis

Concordia Publishing House, St. Louis, Missouri
Copyright © 1978 Concordia Publishing House
Manufactured in the United States of America

Library of Congress Cataloging in Publication Data

Weller, Robert E. 1914—
    Blind—and I see!

    1. Weller, Robert E., 1914— 2. Blind—
Michigan—Biography. 3. Lutheran Church—Clergy—
Biography. I. Title.
HV1792.W44A32   248'.86'0924 [B]   77-13241
ISBN 0-570-03772-0

To the Christian love of the members
of St. John's Lutheran Church, Midland, Mich.;
which refused to be merely an institutional church
or a part of the establishment;

and

To the members of the staff
of the Rehabilitation Center for the Blind
at Kalamazoo, Mich., for their dedication;

and, above all,

SOLI DEO GLORIA

Author's Preface

This little book is simply an account of what results from a blind man lying flat on his back for six weeks. All quotations and historical references are guaranteed inaccurate, also any quotations from the classics. Research is not the strong point of the blind, especially when they are impatient, lazy, and lying flat on their backs.

If this book will encourage the blind, create sympathy for many blind people, and turn some to a realization of God's presence and God's goodness in every time of our need, it will have served its purpose.

Robert E. (Butch) Weller
Midland Hospital
Midland, Mich.
Ash Wednesday, 1976

Contents

Chapter 1
The Thorn in the Flesh

I, the not-so-very reverend Robert E. Weller, the senior pastor of St. John's Lutheran Church in Midland, Mich., was not in a very satisfactory mood. The fourth of October in the year of our Lord 1969 was my fifty-fifth birthday. I really had nothing to grouse about. On the other hand, I could not think of anything to be really jubilant about. My first wife, Clara, was off at St. John's parish school initiating the second and third graders in phonics, arithmetic, and other trivia that present themselves in the curriculum of the lower grades. So I had made my own lunch, the usual sandwich, apple, and bottle of Diet Pepsi. Ah, that "first wife" sort of slipped out, and I'd better explain it. It is simply a whimsical term that I use in introducing my wife to groups of people. It leaves them with sort of a mystery as to whether I have a second wife but still am moving about with my first wife, or whether I am merely vague. It is all really covered by the mention above that I am the not-so-very reverend Robert. Clara says it is evidence of mere wishful thinking.

My lunch having been thoughtlessly and ungratefully relegated to the regions designed for it, I confronted the afternoon—a beautiful fall afternoon—with a sigh and a grimace. There were some routine calls to be made, none so very urgent, but there was no spiritual impulse to send me on my way.

"After all," I argued, making a show of independence against a protesting conscience, "this is my birthday, and since my kith and kin will probably forget all about it, it is only fitting and proper that I should give myself the little present of an afternoon off." Whoever it is that provides justifications in situations like this, and I know it is not always the devil, came forth with the reminder that I was a diabetic, and diabetics need exercise. Exercise is good for their blood sugar. It helps to burn up the sugar that their pancreas does not take care of, even if they are on Diabenes as I am. So I finally overcame all internal opposition by saying to myself simply, "Butch, you need some exercise this afternoon. This is a fine way to spend your birthday. It will be pleasant, and it will be fulfilling a real need." "Butch" is what I call myself when I am really speaking seriously with myself. Butch is an inheritance from my father and from my grandfather who had this same name at college. I used it both at college and at the seminary.

A I rummaged around for a pair of gloves, a saw, an ax, and a spade, I said to myself the old Latin phrase "Sursum corda," which occurs in the liturgy and is translated "Lift up your hearts," and I began to be uplifted just by the thought of going out into the yard and righting some of the wrongs that existed among the shrubbery and other growths. "Sursum corda" reminds me that I should perhaps introduce my cousin Wilfred, who will pop into this little treatise from time to time. He is professor at the Lutheran school, Concordia College, River Forest, Illinois, and knows much of the classics and of many things. He is my fishing companion and one-time bridge partner, and "Sursum corda" recalls a predicament in which he once placed me: We had been having a very exciting bridge hand, he being my partner, and we wanted to get to game and possibly a slam. I had been bidding hearts, and finally he got to game in spades. At this point he happened to mutter "Sursum corda," which could mean "Be joyful. Lift up your hearts, We have it in the bag. We are going to make the game." But since there had been some intimation in the bidding that we should go for a slam, "Sursum corda" could also mean "Maybe you'd better raise me in hearts, and we could do even better." It was a dilemma for

12

me, and finally I chose the wrong course. I raised to a small slam in hearts. This was not what he wanted nor, as the event proved, was it the proper bid, for we went down something like two, doubled and vulnerable. So I can never hear "Sursum corda" without a little bit of a twinge.

But on this October afternoon it *was* "Sursum corda," and I went cheerfully out to do battle with whatever improprieties I might find in the yard. The prospect of physical exercise has always excited me, which may seem strange for a gentleman of the cloth; but it goes way back to my youth. The object upon which I was to exercise my muscles this afternoon was not a football, baseball, golf ball, tennis ball, or even a ping-pong ball but a blameless cherry tree whose only fault was that it had responded well to the pastor's care when he "digged about it and dunged it," to use a Biblical phrase. This cherry tree had grown up from a seed, a volunteer, and it had no place in a yard that was given over only to dwarf trees, dwarf apples, dwarf pears, dwarf apricots, dwarf peaches, and dwarf plums. It was encroaching upon the space of other trees and of the garden itself and though it produced some cherries, the birds got almost all of them.

Laying on like MacDuff with ax and saw and spade, I soon reduced the tree to a pile of brush and a stump about four inches round that protruded about three feet above ground. The brush was carried to the tree lawn, but the stump was a different problem, I dug about it with the spade. I whacked through some roots with the ax. I cut through others with the saw. I dug and dug, and it still maintained its ties with the earth. Finally, by dint of a great deal of heaving and straining and hauling and pulling, and a little more hacking here and a little more whacking there, with one final immense, all-exerting heave, the cherry tree came out with most of its roots, and that task was completed.

Perspiration began to flow, but with it gratification, a feeling of well-being. A more thoughtful person might have paused and asked himself if this love of exertion was perhaps a way of making up for his usual sedentary way of life, but I merely looked about for new fields to conquer and recalled that in the front yard there was another dragon to overcome. This was a Pfitzer evergreen that was in the wrong place and had grown to the wrong size. It either had to be destroyed or relocated, and I determined to move it. Since I wanted to transplant the bush, I first had to dig a cavity in which to replace it. Then, while digging up the bush, I found I could not cut through the roots; I had to take a considerable ball of earth with them. The bush was quite large, and the ball of earth was very heavy. Again there was a session of heaving and straining and hauling and tugging, and finally with a massive effort I lifted the bush with its ball of earth out of the hole, dragged it across the lawn and put it in its new hole, threw some dirt around it and stood back about twenty feet to survey my handiwork. But as I looked at the bush, it seemed to dance. I stared at it, and it would not come into focus. It danced. No, it didn't really dance, it wavered. No, it didn't really waver; I just couldn't get a clear picture of it. I couldn't focus. I looked across the street, and the house there blurred, dimmed, and wavered. I looked up at a tree and saw that it was green, but I couldn't distinguish the individual leaves.

When I realized that there was really something wrong with my eyes, my enthusiasm for my labors oozed out of me like honey out of a comb, and I began to be possessed by a dreadful surmise. I was diabetic, and already years before the optometrist in Rogers City, Mich., had told me that the retina of my eyes was beginning to show the effects of diabetes. He warned me vaguely that this could lead to serious things, but did not tell me precisely what these serious things were. Two years before this birthday activity I had had a brief but frightening experience. I was driving to the hospital, and as I moved along in the car I saw what appeared to be a blob of ink run up the windshield of the car. I reached forward to wipe it away—when I realized it must be on the outside because I could not feel it on the inside. As I came to a corner and looked to the left and to the right, I saw that the blob was not on the windshield but that it was in my eye because it followed wherever I looked. I pulled over to a curb not too far from the hospital and watched as the blob which had run up began to part into various branches until it assumed the form of a leafless tree, a tree in the dead of winter with no foliage, its branches spread starkly against the sky. I did not understand the phenomenon at all but, of course, made my way to my doctor to see what the problem was. My doctor sent me to an eye specialist, an ophthalmologist, Dr. Mesaros, and he told me that I had had a hemorrhage due to my diabetic condition and that a tiny blood vessel in my eye had ruptured. I would have to be careful, to stick to my diet, to do all the things that a diabetic should do and should not do, because there was great danger that such a thing could reoccur. This was only too true. Although the eye cleared up in the space of just a few days, first the twigs, then the branches, and finally the main trunk, yet it was only about six months later that the same things happened in the other eye. This time it was as if a handful of straw or hay had been thrown into my eye. I could see through it, but I could not read or recognize people through it. Again I was frightened, but since the condition cleared up so quickly and my eye seemed to be as good as ever, I refused to be too much concerned. I can't really say whether I had been properly warned by my optometrist in Rogers City or by my ophthalmologist in Midland as to the ultimate consequences of what was happening to my eyes, nor can I really remember being warned against straining, heaving, and lifting. I knew my eyesight would be damaged, but I never thought of such an ultimate thing as a complete loss of sight—blindness!

A few months later, at the end of a New Year's Eve service—the end of a difficult day, the end of a difficult month—I was closing up the church at about 9 o'clock in the evening when suddenly a black blob appeared in my right eye, a large blob, different from the others, with not so many branches and twigs but more and larger projections. This remained for several months before finally fading away. I did not go to the doctor because I presumed I knew what it was all about. I realized, however, that my right eye had been permanently damaged because I could no longer see well enough to read with it.

Now as I looked at the bush but could not focus on it and saw that everything around me was shimmering, hazy, and blurry, all of the things that the doctors told me previously came rushing to my mind. I had never read much about the effects of diabetes upon the eye, but there had been some warnings, and now the significance of the previous hemorrhages came home to me in a new fashion. Was this a precursor of something much worse to come?

I was utterly unprepared for this sort of a development, for only three months before I had had a new pair of glasses made, trifocals in fact, and Dr. Mesaros had said that in the left eye, my good eye, he was able to restore 20/20 vision. I was pleased because with these new glasses I could read the finest print; no footnote was too small for me. But as I looked back, I remembered that sometimes I had difficulty reading in the morning. The eye seemingly had trouble focusing, but this usually passed away after an hour or so. Sometimes, too, I had brief moments of blurred vision. I had heard that this was something that occurred to diabetics as their blood sugar went up and down, so I did not become unduly concerned about it. But now it was another matter.

I gathered my tools and put them away. Then I went into the house and took a shower. I studiously avoided looking at any printed material because this might give me too clear a clue as to what was happening to my eyes. After my shower I stood for a moment in prayer, asking that what was happening to my eyes might be a temporary situation. I went into the living room and lay down on the couch, not yet having the courage to pick up a book and make the ultimate test. After a while I realized I was being

16

cowardly. I would show more confidence in God if I did face this test. So I went over and picked up a Bible and looked at the cover. I could make out the name, "The Holy Bible." I opened the Bible at random and found that I could not distinguish the words or the letters. No matter how hard I squinted, no matter at what distance I held the book from my eyes, I could not focus clearly enough to make out the individual letters. I picked up the newspaper. I could read the headlines; I could read the sub-headlines; but I could not read the text in the columns.

A terrible uneasiness washed over me and I could not concentrate on anything. I peered out the window, closing my left eye, and saw that I could see somewhat clearly with my right eye. But that was the poor eye! I picked up the Bible again. I could not read with my right eye. Now it seemed that my left eye, my good eye, had been chiefly affected by this new crisis. Again I set myself to prayer.

I knew that prayer was something that I could make with boldness, with confidence, and with trust, so I prayed that it might be the Lord's will that my eyesight should be restored shortly. But I also knew that the Lord's ways are sometimes mysterious. I recalled St. Paul's writing in 2 Corinthians 12:7 about "the thorn in the flesh." We do not know exactly what this was. It may have been some sort of eye trouble—some think it was even epilepsy—but it was something that Paul felt came between him and the efficient carrying out of his work, so he prayed to the Lord three times that it might be taken from him. The Lord answered his prayer, but the answer was, "No, My grace is sufficient for you, for My strength is made perfect in weakness." So it is with the thorns in the flesh that come to us, the bodily problems and the sufferings, the aches, the pains, even the blindness. They are the "thorn in the flesh," and sometimes God's grace must be sufficient for us. I prayed with these things in mind and yet with a confidence and trust that a God who has forgiven us all our sins, who has opened the door to eternal life to us, is a

17

God who deals mercifully and gently with us in all of our earthly problems.

In the meditation that went along with my prayer, I realized that vast areas of my life would be affected if this situation did not clear up. It was not merely that I could not enjoy the great outdoors, not merely that I could not enjoy the world of books, not merely that I would be restricted so many ways in my activities, but my very life's work was threatened! Who can conceive of a pastor doing his work when he cannot read? How can a man conduct a church service when he cannot read? How can a man prepare his sermons if he cannot read? How can a man administer to the sick when he cannot see? All of these things flooded in upon me, and I was in a state of shock. Who could doubt that one's very communication with God, which depended so much on reading the Bible, knowing the Bible, searching the Bible, would be lessened by the inability to read? How could one have faith that in such a situation God's strength is made perfect in our weakness?

When Clara came home from school, I had just about finished my prayers and had resolved that I would not reveal the depth of my feelings to her at the present time. She busied herself with supper, and I continued my thinking. I tried not to be too morose or uncommunicative, but it was difficult to keep from giving away the fact that I was not able to read. Since there was no meeting to attend, our evening was a quiet one with the usual discussion of what had happened at school and what I had done during the day. Clara found out that I had cut down the cherry tree and moved the shrub and was pleased. So the evening proceeded into night—a night that was filled with prayers and unrest, but also with hope for tomorrow because again and again I had experienced the blessings of God.

The fifth of October and the beginning of the fifty-sixth year of my life began with foreboding and yet with optimism. I arose early and prepared to carry out the day as usual, made my way to the bathroom, washed, and began to shave. As I looked into the mirror I saw what seemed like a tiny black crow's feather lying horizontally across the upper part of my left eye. This then was what the problem was all about. I looked at the feather with something akin to horror and yet at the same time felt that this was something that the eye had handled before. So I thought, "Another period of waiting, more difficult than the others, but in time everything will be all right." I shaved, got dressed, and my wife and I went off to the church, she to her classroom I to my office. During the course of the morning I worked at such things as I could handle, typing letters and thinking about various things that had to be done.

But about the middle of the morning as I was staring down at my desk, I saw the feather begin to enlarge. It was as if it were bleeding, not in just tiny twigs, but in streams and rivulets that flowed down and formed a big, big blot. This was intolerable. I asked my secretary, Mrs. Hinkle, for Dr. Mesaros' number and called his office. He was in and could see me, so I drove over, all the time noting that the blot in my eye had become so large that I could not tell if it was continuing to bleed. The blot was a little off center, to the side of the nose, but it was huge, and I could see nothing through the eye at all.

The doctor examined me very thoroughly, quietly, and without comment, but afterwards he called me into his special office for consultation, and in a grave voice began to tell me exactly what had happened. He said that I had come to the crossroads, that diabetic retinopathy, which was the technical term for my affliction, had reached a crisis, that I had suffered a blockbuster of a hemorrhage in my good eye, my left eye, and while the right eye was not affected at this time, it was no longer a good eye in any sense of the word. He told me very frankly that diabetic retinopathy now ranked with glaucoma as one of the two greatest causes of blindness among human beings and that I would have to live as carefully as possible, with no lifting, no straining, no exertion, no overwork, and plenty of rest.

Dr. Mesaros also arranged for me to go down to Ann Arbor and see Dr. Wolter, who was the head of the Ophthalmology Department at the University there, to see if I was a candidate for photocoagulation, a technique performed with a xenon arc and later with laser beams. This could possibly preserve my right eye as a useful eye, but the left eye was in such a condition that no photocoagulation could be performed because they would not be able to see what they were doing in the eye. As I sat listening to him, I was full of self-recrimination. How I had indulged myself on my birthday, sawing and digging and hacking, lifting and heaving! And in a sense I may have helped bring this upon myself over the years by not paying enough attention to diet, by the occasional bar of candy, ice cream cone, sundae, peanuts, pie.

Dr. Mesaros told me that at this moment I was already legally blind, and that I really had no business driving, because my right eye would never pass a test. Then he held out a ray of hope. He said, "Sometimes hemorrhages of this kind do indeed clear up, but because of the widespread area which yours covers I fear that the retina will certainly be severely damaged. Nevertheless, we can hold out this hope to you." Finally he said, "Here are some pills which may inhibit bleeding somewhat and help in the absorption of the hemorrhage. I don't really know whether they are very effective, but I think we should try them for a few days. Outside of this, I cannot advise anything except to take it easy, go back to your medical doctor, Dr. Ittner, and have him check again on the blood sugar and on your general condition. General health is important in this case, and it has some effect on the ability of the eye to recover from the hemorrhage."

I shook his hand warmly, thanked him for the information and encouragement he had given me, and went my way. I took the afternoon off, went home, and lay around thinking, meditating, praying, and trying to assess the situation. From time to time I would arise from the couch, go to the front picture window, and stare out at the yard and across the street. I would try to make out new objects with my right eye. I got out my field glasses and found out that I could see much better with my right eye using them. I also found a magnifying glass and could make out some types of print with it. I looked out across the street with my left eye and noticed that I could see color and some objects even from the far left-hand side. I could see cars, although I could not quite identify them, and I could see black and white when I looked at a page, although I could not isolate individual letters. It was encouraging to know that there was still strength in the eye, and I decided to wait and see if the hemorrhage would clear up.

School was over and Clara had come home. This time I told her my problem. She was sympathetic, but shocked, and she too was at a loss as to what we were to do in the days ahead. So we sat down and considered everything. The present situation was not without hope, but there was a question as to whether my good eye would recover. That was a real problem. What then could be done about it? Could I continue in my work as a pastor? For the moment it seemed that I could. I had always preached freely from a detailed outline and felt that I could continue without any difficulty, because I had a good memory. I would be able to memorize texts and even the Gospels and Epistles since I already knew most of them almost by heart. I would have to learn some Collects, some Introits, and Graduals, and would have to avoid or drop out of those services where there were great changes in the liturgy. A great deal of my work involved visiting the sick, visiting in hospitals, counseling, and instructing children and adult classes. These things I felt I could carry on because I could ask the members of the class to read appropriate passages of Scripture, prayers, and things of that kind. But it was with a great deal of doubt and uncertainty that I entered into this new phase of my life.

Chapter 2
Medic, Medic

Dr. Mesaros promptly consulted his connections at the University Hospital in Ann Arbor, and informed me that I had an appointment with Dr. Wolter, the dean of the Ophthalmological Department, for the latter part of October. Ann Arbor was about two hours' drive from Midland, and I could not attempt to drive there. Clara might have taken me, but she was needed at the school. But immediately an elder of St. John's congregation volunteered to take off an afternoon from his job and drive me to the hospital.

By this time I was beginning to gain some confidence in my daily work at St. John's. One of the routine activities was visiting members at the Midland Hospital, a structure which was a kind of cross between a Grecian maze and a rabbit warren, with dead ends, sudden doorways, and hidden staircases. Here I discovered that I had a certain sense of direction and a good memory for any place in which I had been before, and, complicated as the layout of the hospital was, it had been imprinted upon my memory by the four years that I had been active there when my sight was very good. For a while I could even read the numbers on the doorways and was able to find almost any room in the hospital without difficulty.

One annual fall project was the gathering of people interested in joining the church into an adult membership class, and I carried this out in the usual fashion with the assistance of some of the members of the congregation. I also made plans for beginning the Bethel Bible series. My associate, Pastor Brown, and I had attended sessions at

Madison, Wis., in which we learned about the literature and teacher training. Now I began to look about for teachers, candidates for teachers, people with some Biblical background, and people with the spirit to commit themselves to two years of training every Monday night. To make plans for two years and more ahead was a good sign that my self-confidence had been somewhat restored and, cheered by this sort of "business as usual" mood, I looked forward to the trip to Ann Arbor where so many tremendous things have been accomplished in the field of medicine.

We arrived at the University Hospital, and I agreed with my driver to meet him in the lounge after my consultation with Dr. Wolter. The moment I entered the building, I was filled with a feeling of depression. There was a certain coldness to the atmosphere, a certain hustle and bustle which made me wonder whether I would find any help or sympathy, or even understanding, in what seemed to be a mere institution. Someone at the information desk told me to follow the yellow line until I came to an elevator, take that elevator up to the fifth floor, and then follow the yellow line again until it brought me to the offices of the doctor whom I wished to see. So merrily humming "follow the yellow brick road, follow the yellow brick road," from *The Wizard of Oz*, I went more confidently on my way.

While I was seated in the waiting room, the coldness of the hospital was largely dissipated by my meeting the daughter of members of our congregation in Rogers City. She now lived in Alpena, and we immediately began catching up on old times. Then the doctor himself came out to call my name. As I stepped into his office, he greeted me with the words "Herr Pastor." He had looked into my dossier and found out that I was a Lutheran pastor of an age that meant that I would probably be acquainted with the German language. He himself was a German Lutheran, so I responded with "Herr Doktor," and we shook hands. He then repeated the kind of examination

23

that I had had from Dr. Mesaros and also did a few things which seemed new to me.

At last he sat down and told me that he agreed completely with Dr. Mesaros' diagnosis. He said that I had indeed had a massive hemorrhage in my left eye and only time would tell how this would turn out. The right eye had been damaged but was now a candidate for photocoagulation, and he recommended that we set up an appointment so that this could be carried out in order to preserve that eye as much as possible for the future. Dr. Wolter spoke proudly of the xenon arc ray which was used at this time in photocoagulation. He said that many wonderful things had been accomplished by it for many people, and he himself was personally acquainted with the person who had invented the instrument and the technique. A little telephoning, a little consulting of schedules, and an appointment was set for November. Then the doctor and I parted with a cordial exchange of "Auf wiedersehen," and I went to meet my driver, full of warmth, generated by the personality of Dr. Wolter, and hope, generated by his description of the things that had been accomplished through photocoagulation.

After my return to Midland I consulted with Dr. Mesaros again and asked him if there was anything special that I could do to aid my cause. He thought for a moment, then said, "Well, there are some who believe eating fresh raw pineapple is effective in dissolving the hemorrhages that occur in the eyes of diabetic patients." Since he gave this information with a smile, I almost thought of it as a fad or a native remedy, but Clara and I were in the mood to try anything. So during the next month we consumed many and many a fresh pineapple. The Hammerschmidts, members of the congregation, had some contact with Hawaii, and saw to it that we got fresh pineapple right off the plane. The whole procedure reminded me a little of one of my cousin Wilfred's stories in which a witch doctor looks at his patient lying on a cot out in the jungle and finally says, "Well, I am going to dance around him three times more and if that doesn't help we will try sulphanilamide."

About the middle of November I set off for my three-day trip to Ann Arbor, one member driving me down and another to pick me up after the treatment. I still had enough vision that I could enjoy seeing some of the countryside and was particularly impressed by red barns around which the farmers had planted golden fringes of chrysanthemums.

Again I followed "the yellow brick road" to Dr. Wolter's office. Here I found that the first thing I must do was to visit the social worker and have a hospital card made up for myself. Again the cold hospital became a warm place, because the social worker turned out to be a member of one of our churches in the Ann Arbor area, and we were able to converse about people and events we knew in common. Next we met Dr. Gestalter, who was to give me a physical checkup. He put me through all the paces and declared all things to be decent and in order. Then he took me to a special room where there was a large black panel against the wall, and I sat and looked at it while he caused little lights to appear here and there. Apparently the purpose of this was to establish something about my right eye, because I wasn't seeing as well with it as I should. Finally they decided that I had what is called ambliopia in this eye, the failure of the eye to focus properly. I remembered that when I was a boy of 13 or 14, my best friend, Jack Morey, and I used to shoot BB's at a model ship we had made out of toothpicks and modeling clay. I usually used my right eye since I was right-handed, but many of my shots had missed the target. This, apparently, was because of the ambliopia.

The rest of that first day was free, but the next morning I was dressed in appropriate hospital garb and deposited in a corridor on the proper floor. Then it seemed like waiting became the order of the day. Apparently the photocoagulation equipment was used by a number of doctors, and although a schedule had been made out, it was not always possible to tell just how long the equipment would be needed in the case of a given person. But I had received a shot and was in a state of euphoria, so I dreamily contemplated the goings and comings around me, not quite willing to go to sleep, not really taking an interest in the things that went by, and perfectly content to wait my turn. Finally, some time after lunch, Dr. Gestalter and Dr. Wolter appeared, and Dr. Wolter said, "Now it is our turn, and you will see one of the marvels of modern science in the medical field."

Another shot put me in a still more carefree and happy frame of mind, and I thought I talked very engagingly on subjects. The doctors didn't complain about my chatter; probably they had seen this phenomenon in other patients before. I was transferred from my cart to a table over which hung some kind of equipment that was not really like something out of science fiction but was a little bizarre for all of that. My head was cushioned somewhat firmly so that it would remain in place and the doctor said. "You will be conscious of noises and white lights, but there will be no pain whatever. Your eye is desensitized to this treatment, and all you have to do is be patient." I was not only patient, I was friendly; I was loquacious. As Dr. Gestalter and Dr. Wolter worked over me all I was conscious of was a buzzing noise and a white flash, repeated again and again. After perhaps two dozen coagulations, Dr. Wolter said, "Let's have a little more light here, please." Another buzz, crackle, another white light and he continued, "Yes, I see it. I see it by the light of the photocoagulation. Come and look. There is where it is. See, there is a tear in the retina, and this is going to cause us a great deal of difficulty. We will have to go around it as best we can but we cannot touch that part of the eye for fear of doing further damage to the retina. There is a distinct tear in the retina and that is probably why the eye is not as effective as it ought to be."

This was apparently a serious situation, since the doctor was being quite grave about it. But he went on and completed the photocoagulation.

Meanwhile I was feeling quite blithe, and as I recalled Dr. Gestalter's name, I began to burble lines from a German poem, "Der Erlkoenig," which went: "Ich liebe dich, mich reizt deine schoene Gestalt; und bist du nicht willig so brauch' ich Gewalt!" In English it's actually the story of the king of the elves who comes to a young lad and tells him that he wants to take him away from his father. The Elf King says, "I love you. Your fair form entices me, and if you are not willing I will use force." The play was on the German word "Gestalt" and Dr. Gestalter's name. It was foolish; it was silly. But I appealed to Dr. Wolter, "Surely you know 'Der Erlkoenig?'"

He laughed and said, "Yes, I know about it," and I remember feeling a little bit miffed that he did not seem to appreciate my appealing to the classics in such an exalted moment. I suppose, though, that he was busy with more important things.

The flashes of the photocoagulation came to an end and, because of another shot or just general weariness, I drifted off into dreamland and did not come to until just before supper in my little room.

After supper Dr. Wolter came in and in his quiet, dignified, considerate way explained to me that he thought the photocoagulation had been a success, but that the tear in the retina was a problem. It was also a constant danger and could develop in many ways. He could try to stitch the retina together, but in a diabetic this was a hazardous procedure, and since there was no guarantee that it would actually accomplish what was hoped for, he would not recommend it. And so I was free to go home the next morning and I did. Just having had someone try to do something for the eye exhilarated me, and I came home full of enthusiasm and anxious to get back to my work.

Thanksgiving came and I celebrated it by preaching; I celebrated it with my congregation; I celebrated with my wife and such members of my family as were able to come home. We rejoiced in the help that had come to us and in the support of our congregation. Though nothing had been done about my left eye, since no photocoagulation could occur until it had been cleared up, I was still optimistic that it would come around. The doctor had said there was every possibility that this might happen, and we had confidence that the grace of God would bring it about. So we went on with our lives with zest and vigor.

At this point, I should say a word about the problems of a wife in such a situation. Clara expressed only compassion, sympathy, and interest, but I know she worried about security, the future, and much more. She assumed care of the checkbook, which had been my task. She worked with our income tax, which is quite complicated for someone in the ministry. She took over driving the car and paying the bills. It is difficult for a person going blind to appreciate how much work he lays upon the person who lives with him, and at the same time it is difficult for the sighted person to realize just how far blindness has proceeded. The sighted person will tend to say that something is "over there," pointing in a direction that the blind person cannot see. For Clara and me this became a growing problem because, though my eyesight was stable for a while, it soon grew worse and eventually I was to lose it completely. The time was to come when she would put food on my plate; then say that the meat was at six o'clock, the peas at three o'clock, the potatoes at nine o'clock, and the salad at twelve o'clock. It is difficult for both blind and sighted persons to become accustomed to such directions and both must make some serious adjustments.

About two weeks after the photocoagulation, the real jolt came. I was lying on the couch, thinking about the coming Sunday and the text I was going to use. I lay in a position that enabled me to gaze out of the window, and I reached for something that was lying on the floor. This movement required some exertion and when I regained my position on the couch and looked back out the window, I saw the dreaded thing again—a trickle of blood, the little twigs and branches beginning to grow in my right eye. So the photocoagulation had not been completely successful and this was a terrible blow. Now no reading was possible even with the reading glass, now no driving was possible. And for a few days I felt like the man in the nursery rhyme: "All the king's horses and all the king's men couldn't put Humpty Dumpty together again." Everything seemed to fall apart.

I remembered the words of our Lord which tell us that we should build upon a rock, not upon the sand. "He who hears these words of Mine and does them I will liken him to a man who built his house upon the rock, and the rains came and the floods descended, and they could not shake this house because it was built upon a rock." I had in a sense built part of my house upon the sand, at least the outbuildings. I had depended a great deal on what was going to be done for me at Ann Arbor, what the medics could do for me. But I'd also built upon the rock. I had committed my future to God, to Christ, and I knew that His promise was, "I am with you always even to the end of the world." As Psalm 23 puts it, "Surely goodness and mercy shall follow me all the days of my life." I prayed again and though I knew that prayer did not always bring the result that we expect, I also knew that it always brings God's answer and God's help.

Christmas was drawing near and with it the ultimate sign of God's love—the gift of His only-begotten Son to the world. The God who thus goes all out for man is not going to leave a Christian unattended, uncomforted, and unhelped in times of crisis. It might be that God did not want me to continue in the ministry, but my life would continue and so it was a time for faith. Surely faith must show itself most strongly when there seems to be no answer to a prayer.

In my distress my mind reverted to the last call I had made before I finally decided that I could not drive any longer. This was to an old woman of 80, who was staying with one of her children over in Bridgeport. I only had to pass one traffic light to reach Bridgeport and since I had been calling on this lady for a long time and had some success in dealing with her, I decided to go. The woman suffered from hardening of the arteries and was now living fifty years in the past, which was a very great trial for her son and daughter-in-law. When people spoke to her in English, she frequently burst into fits of rage, threw things, and berated them. I discovered that she had come to America from Germany as a young mother, and when she reached Ellis Island, officials found out that her child had chicken pox. The child was removed from her and she, who had not as yet any command of the English language, was utterly confused and thought that her child was being taken from her forever. Although the child was returned about two weeks later when the illness was over, she never forgot her frightening experience and now associated anyone who spoke to her in English with the officials on Ellis Island. When I spoke to her in German, she seemed more content and told me that her father would be returning from work in a few hours and that she would like me to meet him. Of course her father had been dead for fifty years, but she was living in the happier past she remembered in Germany. On the whole we got along very well and when I spoke the Lord's Prayer, she was with me all the way. I even got to the point where I could commune her; and when I did so in German, she understood everything I said.

So it was to this old woman that I made my last call alone, because when I came to Bridgeport and approached the light, I could not tell whether it was red or green. I stopped and immediately a long line of cars began honking behind me. I assumed that I should go ahead and I did, but it frightened me so much that I realized that I should never drive the car again.

As I contemplated the likelihood that I would have to give up the making of calls which had been so much a part of my ministry, I looked back over the past thirty years. I thought of my beginnings in Oklahoma and the trips out to Gowen from McAlester. Gowen was a ghost mining town and in it lived a family with whom I had spent considerable time. The old man had consumption, yet he still labored to dig a few tons of coal out of the mine and sell it. One evening as I walked with him to the services we were going to hold in the American Legion Hall, a very modest building with stone walls and a dirt floor, he began to sing. I recognized the old Lutheran chorale "Allein Gott in der Hoeh sei Ehr'," "All glory be to God on high." I asked him where he had learned this song and he said, "Oh, when I was in Austria. I was a German who lived in Austria, and I sang in a children's choir over there in Vienna." I realized then that he had been a member of the well-known Vienna Boys' Choir, but also that he did not realize how famous this choir had since become. I continued to minister to him and buried him when he died. His family moved to Flint, Mich., and after many years I had resumed contact with them and was happy to learn that they were still members of the Lutheran church, especially since I had thought at the time that my brief stay in Oklahoma had borne no fruit at all.

I remembered the years when I had been pastor in Gospel Center in Cleveland, Ohio. There we reached out to people on welfare, on relief, to the handicapped, the blind, the crippled, to anyone that the church could not reach. So many of these had to be visited, and I remembered how many of them had begged me to be sure to visit them at the hospital so they would not be kept there without a friend to speak for them.

I thought of my ministry in Normal, Ill., where I had also found elderly people who became my friends and whom I was able to console with the Gospel and with prayer, though visiting them often required long trips out into the country.

I thought of my ministry in northern Michigan. There was an old man who listened to our radio broadcasts from Rogers City, and whom I finally sought out although he lived about thirty miles away. I found him in the backwoods, far off the state highway, far off the county road, on a little lane in a humble house where he lived with his mentally retarded daughter, who spent much of her time sitting and rocking in a chair. She would not meet visitors, and her father said he had trouble keeping her dressed, but she took care of the house and cooked for him as well as anybody could. I remember communing him in the quietness of his house in the midst of winter, when he was practically shut off from civilization.

I thought of the many people whom I now knew in Midland, and it was with a pang that I realized that if I had to give up my ministry all of this was a part of the past and I could only dream about it. But I did not sufficiently know the goodness of God and the love of the people of St. John's church; only later did I learn it.

Christmas came, and with it all the consolation and joy that fills the Christian heart with the announcement that Christ, the Savior, is born. The family got together, and my eye even improved enough so that we could play some bridge. We also enjoyed opening the packages from our daughter and son-in-law in the Philippines and looking at some of the pictures they had sent us. In general, we had all the fellowship, the love, and the joy that comes to Christian people when they remember the birthday of Jesus Christ, their Savior.

The most important gift I received was from my sister Dolly, a widow who had worked her way through various stages of education until she had become a nurse. Then she took a degree and finally became dean of the School of Nursing at the University at Marquette, Mich. She conceived the idea of sending me a tape recorder for Christmas. It was a Craig model and admirably suited for use by a blind person because it had only one control lever, instead of the usual five push-buttons featured by many other tape recorders. I soon found what a valuable tool this was for the ministry of a blind person. Clara could record the Gospels, Epistles, Collects, Introits, Graduals, and all the parts of the Lutheran liturgy that changed each Sunday on the tape, and I could memorize them at my leisure during the week. The recorder became my constant companion (in fact I am using it now). I also found that the State Library was an invaluable source of material, not only for further education but also for recreation. It supplied many titles both on cassettes and also on records and would also provide a record player and a tape player for those who desired them, with all postage involved free of charge.

A new year, 1970, thus started on an optimistic note, especially when a little cartoon appeared on the bulletin board of the church one day. It depicted a motorcycle driven by a beautiful girl, while in the sidecar sat a pastor in his full clericals, his stole waving in the breeze. Beneath was the legend, "Register here in order to volunteer to drive for the Pastor." Immediately scores of names were added and from that day to the present I have never lacked a driver, male or female, young or old, to take me wherever I want to go—in the town, out into the country, to nearby cities such as Bay City and Saginaw, or even to farther off places such as Lansing, Ann Arbor, and Detroit. This solved my problem of mobility. I could go wherever I wanted to. I could visit nursing homes; I could visit the hospital; I could visit people anywhere in the parish. A fine relationship grew up between the drivers and myself because they were not simply drivers. They became assistant ministers. They helped me administer communion; they helped me with prayers and Scripture readings; they expressed their own comfort and consolation to the sick; and they joined in conversations in a lively and interesting way. This has been one of the most wonderful supports the congregation could give me, and I never cease to appreciate it.

At the beginning of 1970 we also had to get our Bethel Bible series under way. Eighteen teachers were champing at the bit, as it were, to get ahead with this project in which they had become very much interested. All had committed themselves to study for two years and then to teach for a year. We were ready to go when again I received a jolt as far as my eyesight was concerned. This is always the problem with the diabetic. Once he has had a hemorrhage, it seems only a matter of time before another hemorrhage or some other unhappy development must be faced. While we were making our plans to go ahead with the Bethel Bible series, I arose one morning, looked in the mirror to shave, and could hardly distinguish my face. At first I thought it was just early morning drowsiness and bleary-eyedness, but after shaving and washing I realized it wasn't this at all. Something had happened to my eye. I had learned my lesson, and I called the doctor's office immediately and was told to come down. So someone transported me, and the doctor immediately went through his usual examination. When he was finished, he shook his head and said, "Remember the tear in your retina that Dr. Wolter discovered? One corner of it has curled up, and that's why you are unable to see with any degree of clarity. I must put you in the hospital at once so that, if possible, we can get the flap of the retina to lie down flat again. I can't even contemplate operating on an eye such as yours, first because you are a diabetic and second, because the situation in the eye is so delicate that I don't think any form of operation would be helpful."

So I was bundled off to the hospital, and, since no other room was available, was placed in the intensive care ward. This is a place for people who are very ill indeed. While I was unhappy enough because I had to lie flat on my back without even a pillow underneath my head and had been given a sedative to keep me that way, I could hear the groans, cries, shrieks, and complaints of the people around me, and had to acknowledge that I did not suffer actual physical pain. I remained in the intensive care ward for only one night, but in the hospital for four days. At the end of this time Dr. Mesaros came to me and said, "Well, I have good news for you."

It was hard for me to refrain from saying, "Well, it's about the first good news that I have ever received from you." But he did have good news: the retina had flattened out. When I got up and looked around I could see a little bit better than I had when I entered the hospital, but my eye had not returned to its former strength and my field of vision had been cut by perhaps 25 percent. When I looked straight ahead I could see, but there was a sort of crinkling in my eye. The effect was to make everything look like a photograph that had been crumpled and imperfectly flattened. This condition improved a little in the following months, but my eye never regained its former power, and the hopes which I had had for carrying on in almost a normal way were dashed.

Meanwhile, the doctor stated that he felt one of the reasons why my eye was responding as it did was because I spent too much time at my work, pushed myself too hard. Now I would have to take it easy, or I would bring about an even more rapid dissolution of the eye. He suggested that I work half days, so we set up a new plan whereby I did only spend half days on things like making calls, visiting hospitals, nursing homes and things of this kind. I spent the mornings just in reading, listening to tapes. The evenings were for attending meetings. Thus I cut down my workload by at least 30 percent, if not by 50 percent.

Nevertheless, we wanted to go ahead with the Bethel Bible series, and I felt that I ought to ask Pastor Brown to take over under these circumstances. He had gone with me to Madison to take the two-week course offered there. When I approached him, though, he hedged and said that he had not really gotten much out of the presentations at Madison, and felt that he did not want to take this upon himself. So I reconsidered whether I could carry on a successful training period, perhaps with Clara's help in reading the lessons for me each week and relying on my general knowledge of the Scriptures.

As I pondered this, two fine women of the congregation came to my assistance. One was Mrs. Lois Reed who said she would place the lessons on tape from week to week so that I would be able to study the material at my leisure. This was such a welcome offer that I not only accepted it but came very close to kissing her in gratitude. The second woman, Mrs. Vi Friedrich, said that since she was going to be a teacher, she thought it would benefit her to sit down with me on Monday mornings and go through the lessons with me. She would be willing to devote two or three hours every Monday morning for at least two years. She received a handshake and a pat on the back.

With the help of these two ladies and my wife, and the full cooperation of everybody else, we began the two-year study of the Bible as it is outlined in the Bethel Bible series. This became a most wonderful experience. The eighteen people whom we had chosen fit together beautifully. There was fellowship; there was laughter; there was repartee; there was argument; there was sharing; there was everything that one could wish, and the spirit of fellowship, the "esprit de corps" that developed was tremendous to behold. A fine relationship grew up between me and these teachers, and they were responsible for the fact that eventually we had 250 people coming to Bible class on Wednesday night. This continued for a good long time, and the program is still being carried on after these several years.

While I devoted a lot of energy to the work of the congregation, I was also mindful, as a blind person always is, of every advance in science that might be helpful. *The Reader's Digest* had published an article which said that an adaptation of the TV principle had been used to create an instrument to aid the blind. A small TV camera was so mounted that it would read a small paragraph of print, then transmit this electronically to a large television screen, thus magnifying the print many times. Many people were able to read by means of this instrument. I was intrigued and immediately investigaed, sending for literature from the address given in *The Reader's Digest*. I found out that the parts would cost some $500, and we thought of ordering them and asking a number of electronic experts in the congregation to put the mechanism together. However, before we invested any money, Clara and I decided to drive down to Kalamazoo one summer day and find out just how the machine operated. There were a few of these machines in the state and one was at the Rehabilitation Center for the Blind in Kalamazoo. One of the girls there, who had limited vision, used it to enable her to do secretarial work. We went down and were permitted to see the instrument and use it. But to my dismay, I found that my eyes had deteriorated to such an extent that even with the magnification provided on the television screen I could only make out occasional letters here and there and could not really read with any facility.

This was a disappointment. At the same time it is the sort of thing that a blind person learns to cope with. He finds an article in *Time* magazine about some new advances in treating the eyes of the blind and is immediately intrigued by it. Or he gets a clipping from some friend about somebody who has had special photocoagulation treatment and has been wonderfully improved. This sort of thing goes on and on, and the blind person is always ready to the point of gullibility to believe anything that holds any promise at all. Some magazines announced that electrodes, planted in the backs or foreheads of blind persons and properly connected, have enabled the persons to pick up outlines of the things before them. But none of these things seemed to apply to a pastor who had to do a lot of reading. So even though all of them were investigated—and I sometimes made trips to Dr. Mesaros' office to ask him about a new technique that I heard about, he always regretfully said he was afraid this would not be helpful to me in my situation.

During the early months of 1970 I made at least two more trips to Ann Arbor to visit Dr. Wolter and see what his final decision might be. On what turned out to be the last trip, Clara went with me, because I found I could no longer follow "the yellow brick road" by myself. So we went up to see Dr. Wolter together. He received me graciously and kindly, as always, and was particularly pleased to meet Clara. He again made an examination, a somewhat cursory one, but he did take out red and green flashlights to see if I could distinguish the two colors. I could, and he said that this was a good sign that the retina was still reacting very strongly to anything it came in contact with and that behind these hemorrhages there was no doubt an eye that still was useful and valuable. But he said that he did not know of any way to remove the hemorrhages. When I remarked that some had suggested that the vitreous humor of the eye, the liquid, could be exchanged for some other medium, he said that work had been done along this line with some success, but in the case of diabetics it was a project with little hope for success. He warned us that while we could go many places and find doctors who would operate on my eyes, the chances of any beneficial results were almost nil, and he advised against permitting anyone to do such a thing. My eye would clear itself by God's blessing, on its own, but medical science would not be able to accomplish it. His final word to us was, "You are Christian people, and my best advice to you is to go home, be patient, and pray." And so we did.

At this point it seemed as if I had suffered some almost irremediable reverses. I was no longer able to drive; I was no longer able to read. What little sight I had was failing. On the other hand, my work was still going on. I was able to function at an almost normal pace, and I recognized that really my trust had not been in the medical profession, which had now said, "We can do nothing for you," nor in the ability of my body to recuperate naturally. No, my trust had always been that God would find some way, would bless me, and answer my prayers in His own way. I was to find that He had already chosen a way, and His medium would be the Christian faith and love of the members of St. John's church, who rallied about, showed support, encouraged, and accepted my ministrations. I could not but recognize that God wanted me to continue in the ministry and that my ministry was going to be blessed.

A great forward step had been taken already by the people of St. John's in accepting the ministrations of a blind pastor. Sometimes people do not realize how hesitant they are about approaching a blind person. They shy away, unsure of how to talk to him or what to say, and so they avoid contact completely. This increases the isolation of the blind person who cannot seek out persons for himself. He depends upon people to talk to him, and he tries to hold them by his interest, by his appreciation for their taking time to speak to him. The people of St. John's, seeing my blindness come upon me very slowly, had not been overwhelmed by it but had grown gradually accustomed to it and were perfectly at ease in my presence, blind though I was.

Chapter 3

One Hundred and Fifty Pairs of Eyes

By Easter 1970, I had been essentially blind for six months, and I had remembered not only what the Scripture says about "Ask and it shall be given you; seek and ye shall find," but also Dr. Wolter's advice: "Go home and pray." My prayers were frequent and sometimes very insistent, but no answer seemed to be given until one day when I was in an unusually bright and intelligent mood I suddenly realized that God *had* answered my prayer in a most unusual way. He had not restored my independence; He had not returned my reading ability or driving ability; but He had done something much more wonderful. He had given me one hundred and fifty pairs of eyes that I could use at any time and any place!

One day I asked the lady who was in charge of making up my weekly driving schedule how many names we had on the list. She counted them, and they came to one hundred and fifty. Besides this, Mrs. Brown—wife of Pastor Brown—had begun to establish a readers' list and this involved quite a number of names also. So I was blessed with the eyes of all kinds of people, young, old, teenagers, people in school, people out of school, people retired, people at work, widows, widowers—all came to my aid. Once I suggested that I ought to pay each of them for their services. This was declined with ridicule. I felt, though, that since the congregation still gave me a car allowance, which we only used in part for Clara's driving and driving me about, I ought to do something for these people. I finally compromised by sending so much a month to the women's group of the church, and they did with it as it pleased them. With this monthly expenditure and a yearly party for the drivers and readers, my conscience was cleared.

These same people often told me that their jobs as drivers and readers were not only a source of satisfaction, but also a source of spiritual growth. As they read to me, they became acquainted with materials which they would not otherwise have known. They went out on calls with me and had that distinct feeling of satisfaction which comes to a person when he has put himself out for others who are in great need. People in nursing homes, for example, are in great need, not generally of food or clothing or things of that kind, but simply for friendship, for reassurance, for the support of their faith in Christ through regular devotions. The drivers saw these things. They were impressed, their own lives were changed, and they became more effective workers in the church because of the experience they had with me. I must confess, too, that having a series of drivers was a wonderful way for me to make more calls than ever before. I would no longer come home for lunch on a given day and, as I did on that birthday when I lost my eyesight, change my mind about the afternoon's agenda. I was now planning a schedule a week in advance and so avoided these temptations. My drivers would come punctually at 2 p.m., when we would start making calls, and end generally at 5:30 p.m. The same thing was true in the morning. I could have skipped going to the office many mornings, but there was my reader waiting for me at nine o'clock, and it became a routine which caused me to flourish and caused them to be blessed.

It may seem ridiculous for a blind person to give directions to people, and yet I was able to do this for my drivers and on individual occasions to other people. Sometimes my drivers were hesitant about taking me certain places, but I assured them that I knew the way. In

41

fact, I was quite dictatorial about what roads they should take and what streets they should follow to get to the place where I wanted to be. I recall one day a lady driver of mine asked me where I wanted to go. I said, "Let's go to the hospital." I was busy thinking about something as we went on our way, and when I became aware again of where we were, I noticed that she was downtown. I said, "I'm sorry. You must have misunderstood me. I didn't want to be downtown. I wanted to be at the hospital."

She said, "I can't find the hospital from the church, but if I go downtown first, then I can find it from there."

Now besides being a mile out of her way, the kind of thing that struck me as inept, I realized I needed to be more explicit in my directions. As a result I became very bossy and gave my drivers orders.

Another day when I was taking my constitutional around the church, a man drove up and asked me for directions. I gave him these exactly, but after he saw my cane he said, "Oh, sorry."

I said, "Don't be sorry. The directions are good. You'll find your way." And so off he went.

The truth is a blind person makes use of his memory much more than the ordinary person does. When the blind person goes somewhere and has any expectation at all that he might go there again, he carefully marks the streets and the crossings and the lights so that he can make the trip on his own if the occasion should arise. Even in the matter of telephone numbers I began to memorize. It was, after all, embarrassing to ask one's secretary for a number and then to find the line busy. Then you would ask her for the same number a few minutes later, and if the line was still busy, you would have to ask a third time. I found out that you can remember a great many numbers if you set your mind to it. People who are sighted are not pressed to do this, and they think they could not because their memory is not good. But memory can be trained.

A blind person also trains his memory so that he knows where he has placed things and can pick them up later.

Sometimes, of course, one is confounded by cleaning women and housewives who change things about, saying, "I didn't move a thing." But actually they moved things six or seven inches out of place, and I knew the difference. Clara would often say, "It's just where you left it," but this is not practically true for a blind person unless the object really hasn't been moved at all.

My drivers became of real assistance to me in many other ways too. When I wanted to administer communion to a sick person or a shut-in, the driver would prepare the elements. At first I tried to distribute the elements, but because of my blindness it was a little bit difficult, especially when the sick person was not able to cooperate very well. So in recent years, the driver always gives the bread and the wine to the communicant while I speak the essential words. This may not be considered perfectly kosher in some areas of the church, but I think it is completely defensible, even if the driver is a woman.

Drivers also would carry a little portfolio with all kinds of devotional books in it: *Portals of Prayer, The Good News,* and *Strength for the Day.* In addition there was sometimes a coloring book for a child or some kind of literature that was suitable for a child, some Sunday bulletins for people who had missed church, and a booklet for new mothers called *The Magnificat.*

Generally I knew about where I would be calling and sometimes realized that a particular call was rather delicate and could be conducted better by the pastor alone. When this was the case, the drivers very accomodatingly would sit in their cars and read or listen to the radio until I finished my call and came out, with head sometimes bloodied, but unbowed.

There were constant exchanges between my drivers and readers and me, which made our relationship very comfortable. Sometimes I would say to my driver, "Let's stop at the bar in the next block." With a somewhat shocked expression, the driver would say, "Do you really thing we ought to?" and I would assure her that it was

43

perfectly all right. So we would move on to the next block and I would point out the bar, which was a dairy bar. Because of this little experience, the drivers were continually telling each other and their friends that the pastor had dropped in with them at a bar that afternoon. Of course, since I was on a diabetic diet, ice cream was a "no-no" for me along with candy, cake, pie, and a considerable number of other things. Some of my drivers were so intent on seeing to it that I kept to my diet, that they would refuse to stop at the bar even if it was the dairy bar. "You don't need those calories. Those sweet things are not good for you," they informed me. And they were right.

The annual banquet became a hilarious sort of affair. It began on a rather formal note with a speaker who had been a pastor in Africa, followed by a menu of chicken and swiss steak served by the ladies of the congregation. Next there came singing, reminiscences about the past year's experiences, and fun-poking at some of the incidents. I acted as master of ceremonies and tried to keep things running smoothly and quickly. There were also drawings for door prizes for men and for women, for the best driver, the best woman driver, and the best man driver, and finally a beauty contest which was also settled by drawing a number out of a hat. One year, the group rebelled at this way of deciding who was the most beautiful driver, so the next year when we happened to have another blind person as a guest at the banquet, I invited her to select the most beautiful woman. She went from place to place talking to the ladies and finally said, "I like this one. I like her voice."

At later banquets of this kind I had an opportunity to pass on information that I had learned at the Rehabilitation Center for the Blind. There is, for example, a proper and improper way of leading the blind. The proper way is to let the blind person take hold of your right elbow. This leaves him free to carry his cane in his right hand—if he has a cane with him—and to follow you very carefully about half a step behind. When you make a turn, he is able to follow it easily because he has hold of your elbow. When you come to a narrow place when you cannot go abreast, the proper signal is for the sight guide to hold this arm directly in back of him so that the blind person is forced to recognize this and walk in the footsteps of the person who is doing the guiding.

One must be careful of stairways, and the good sight guide pauses so that the blind person knows he is going up the stairs or down the stairs. Then he begins to walk again and the blind person follows him just one pace behind. A regular rhythm should be kept up and when the sighted person gets to the top step, he should pause. The blind person catches this and does not then paw around with his foot high in the air trying to find another step.

I used to claim I had touched so many right arms that I could tell within two pounds how much the person weighed. This was, of course, a big lie but some were quite impressed by it and, if they were a little overweight, they would gasp and not want to know any more about it. But if they were of normal weight, they would oftentimes press for an estimate. Actually I could not gauge my guide's weight within fifty pounds, but I would select a weight which I guessed was at least ten or fifteen pounds below what the person actually weighed. This proved a tactful way of beating a retreat when one opened his big mouth too far.

The name "reader" for those people who served me in the morning in the office was a kind of a misnomer, because sometimes their activities included no reading at all. They corrected papers, graded and filed them, helped clean out my file drawers so I could make a little sense out of them, and, when necessary, took me to the barber or to do a little shopping, to the ophthalmologist and to the medical doctor. At times they would have to step out while a person came in for counseling.

One thing is certain: the people who send out junk mail, even the people who write from the church headquarters or district offices do not realize how much time has to be spent in reading their materials. As a blind person, I found it very difficult to keep up with them. Even with a reader of the best goodwill we could not make progress enough, and many a church press release, many a pamphlet, many a piece of literature was simply dumped in the trash barrel.

The readers also had the responsibility of helping me check out my Sunday sermon text. They would read it in several versions so that I understood it, and they would then help pick hymns, make up the order of service, and turn it all over to the secretary. Once in a while they even had to be witnesses at a baptism or a wedding.

The congregation's desire to show its love for the pastor and their confidence in his work showed itself in another way which was most encouraging. I had celebrated thirty years of my ministry in the fall of 1969, and at the beginning of 1970 the congregation resolved secretly to hold a special service in honor of my thirty years of service and also to gather a purse for me. They consulted with my wife, and she got them pictures of all kinds. A display was made in the lounge of the church. I had no inkling of what was going on. One Sunday afternoon, Clara and I were invited out for supper by some members of the congregation. After supper they said, "Let's go over to the church for a moment. There is something that we want to see there."

When we got to the church, the parking lot and the side streets were packed with cars, and I knew something was up, but I still had no idea of what it was. Then I found out. Clara and I were seated near the altar as guests of honor. (Our church is in the round and it is a little bit difficult to know where to seat special guests.) The president of our district was there to speak, and the church was packed with a large group of pastors from the area, many members of my congregation and people from surrounding congregations. One of the most surprising things was that the choir of my former congregation in Rogers City turned out and made the 150-mile trip just to attend this service and sing with the St. John's choir.

After the service there were refreshments and everybody could look at the pictures which included some of me as an infant in, well, what my cousin Wilfred would call "puris naturalibus." At the end of the proceedings, a check for almost a thousand dollars was presented to me.

These special acts of love and consideration and support were wonderfully encouraging, and I was slow in realizing that the even greater thing my congregation did for me was simply to forget that I was blind. As I mentioned before, many people shy away from a blind person initially because they do not know how to handle him. The congregation at St. John's never really had to deal with this problem consciously because my blindness came on so slowly. While they were for a long time expecting their poorly sighted pastor to regain his sight, when it disappeared completely, it did not seem to change their attitude toward him at all. In general, this is the chief responsibility which the public owes to blind people too, and I felt that St. John's congregation was showing something to the rest of the world.

The problem that most people have with blind persons is the problem of the Christian pastor too. I could sense that while my good friends and classmates came up and said, "Hello" to me at conferences, they didn't know how to carry on a conversation with me. They were apparently afraid of stepping on my toes, of offending me, of bringing back some memory that might be unhappy, and it almost seemed sometimes as if they were avoiding me. I am sure that this was not the case, but they had to learn to become accustomed to me, and eventually did so by merely following the golden rule, loving their neighbor as they loved themselves. The pastors of the district soon even restored me to my honorary position as after-dinner speaker to the ladies who had prepared meals for the pastors, a task I'd always enjoyed.

Soon after the congregation had strengthened me with this thirtieth anniversary celebration, the chairman of the conference realized that it was time to call upon me again.

He came up to me when I was halfway through the stew, which gave me just a few scattered minutes to think of something to say. I got up and began by saying, "There is one thing that is always a little difficult for the speaker for the conference and that is a tendency to stare at certain women more than at others. I do not want to say this definitely, but it might be because he thinks some are prettier than others. With me, you don't have to worry about such favoritism. You all look beautiful to me. You're all tall, statuesque, blondes or brunettes, and I know this to be a fact."

After some laughter, I continued: "You have served us a wonderful meal today. For me it was an especially exciting meal. I filled my plate blindly from the various bowls before me, a spoonful of this, a spoonful of that, and when I finally sat down and thrust my fork into something it was really a matter of excitement. What was I getting? It felt slippery. What might it be? I thrust it into my mouth, and it was an onion. I tried again. What is this? A piece of potato? No, it's a piece of meat. And so I go on, each forkful a new adventure in enjoying the culinary art, and I say to you ladies, all of these things that I tasted, each of which came to me so blindly, was excellent. There wasn't a single off-taste spoonful in the whole stew, and so we thank you ladies, not only for being so beautiful and for being so patient, but also for being such excellent cooks and satisfying us to such a wonderful extent with your hospitality." And so I got back into the ranks of after-dinner speakers.

Perhaps this chapter is mistitled "One Hundred and Fifty Pairs of Eyes." It's true that these special people rendered very special services to me, but all 1,500 communicants, all 2,200 souls of St. John's church did their part. They came to church; they contributed to the church; they had fellowship with one another; they accepted me. And they went along with the difficult moments too. There were times when I could not be available on short notice to read a Scripture selection;

there were times when the doctors told me to take it easy, and I had to go on half days for a while; there came times when I had to be hospitalized again. But the congregation simply blossomed under this adversity, and the immense number of calls that I made on the sick, the shut-ins, those in hospitals, and those new in town helped to break down any feeling that a blind person could not be the pastor of a congregation. Because people saw me active and heard my messages in their own homes, it was not difficult for them to come to the church. I stood openly at the door and greeted them as they went out, recognizing many of their voices, calling them by name before they were able to introduce themselves to me, and in general putting them at their ease as they put me at my ease. It was my whole congregation, as well as members of surrounding congregations who also helped, that made all this possible. Without all of these people I would not have had a second chance in the ministry; with them I could begin to see that the greatest things in my ministry were yet to come.

Chapter 4
Counterattack

The one hundred and fifty pairs of eyes that God had given me in response to my prayers soon began to shape my ministry into new, yet old, forms. The morning readers almost dictated regular office hours, because we had to set up a schedule at least a week in advance as to who would be reading on a particular day. This regular schedule enabled me to keep abreast of my mail and also helped me set aside time for consultations with troubled people, people who had marriage problems or who wanted to be married, and people who for some reason or other wanted simply to talk things over with the pastor. At first, when I was supposed to be taking it easy, the readers had come to the house, but as that period passed they would simply pick me up, take me to the church, and work with me there from 9 till 12. Then they would return me to my home for lunch. After a while, though, I realized that we could save them some driving if I would come to the church at 7:30 with my wife. In her capacity as parish school teacher she was to be there at 7:30 to take part in the morning devotions which the teachers held for themselves in the little chapel next to my office. I soon found that it was good for me to take part in this chapel exercise too. And I established good contact with the teachers and knew what was going on in their field simply by being there at 7:30 in the morning.

Before the reader came then at 9 o'clock, I could type letters, devote myself to thinking about the text for the following Sunday, or bring along my tape recorder and memorize certain things that I wanted to use for the next

Sunday's service or some class. So I was able to add more than an hour and a half to my morning, a real advantage, because a blind person simply needs more time to do certain things. He can't just sit down and quickly read through a few paragraphs of a magazine article to get what he wants. It takes him time to have someone read it to him. He also must sit down and think things out and, not having printed material before him, this also takes time, more time than a sighted person requires. So I was very happy to have this additional time to work on various things in the early morning hours.

I took a long lunch hour, not only because I had to make my own meals but also because this gave me some opportunity for reading tapes which had come to me, tapes from the State Library for the Blind or that somebody had made for me of a meeting they had attended. This was both informational reading, study, and sometimes mere recreation.

The prompt arrival of my afternoon drivers at 2 p.m. meant that no time was lost getting to work in the afternoon. I discovered that work in the hospital could be intensified, calls could be made every other day and followed up in a way which had not been possible before. Many people, after being released from the hospital, spend long hours in illness and weakness at home, or sometimes, if the doctor so directs, in a nursing home. Now we were able to follow these people wherever they went. I realized that entering nursing homes meant opportunitites to offer services to many people, to bring prayer and Scripture to people who were not being served by any minister at all. This expanded our work so that soon we were active in several nursing homes in Midland as well as a number in Saginaw, Bay City, and other towns in the surrounding area.

The driving schedule soon had to be drawn up to include evening calls, an important matter in a parish, because there are many people who cannot be reached except when they come home from work. At the same time there are a great many meetings that are held in the church in the evenings, and it is sometimes difficult to find enough evening hours to make the calls that have to be made. When I had driven myself, I would almost always leave the house soon after supper and make a call or two on my way to a meeting. However, I felt that I could not impose upon my drivers in this way, so we made the best possible use we could of any evening hours that we had. The driver would come at 6:30, and we would make calls until perhaps 9:30 or 10 o'clock on those evenings which were otherwise free. We also found out that certain evenings, such as Fridays, were not good for making calls on people, but that Saturday afternoons were sometimes very good. So, one way or another, we were able to make the calls which are necessary for a pastor to make in a large congregation in a populous city.

My drivers, readers, and everybody in the congregation had simply assumed all along that any day now Pastor's eyesight would begin to improve, but I knew that there was no improvement. In fact, there was only deterioration, and I could not conceal it. For example, I could no longer recognize people and had to apologize for this. As I depended more and more on the sound of their voices, I had to ask them to speak up so that I could identify them in this way. Without much discussion, the assumption finally seemed to be made that Pastor was not going to get his eyesight back, and nobody made much of a fuss about it. The drivers kept on signing up; the readers kept on signing up; and the work was done quite efficiently. It was just a new state of affairs with which everybody went along. Sometimes after a call, I would ask the drivers for their impression of a certain person or a certain situation, because something in the background was not clear to me. I sometimes even went so far as to ask if the house was well kept, if it looked as if they had sufficient funds to operate their household, how many children were around, and things of that sort. My drivers were invaluable for the impressions they gave me of the places we visited.

My confidence also grew in conducting the services, and I felt quite at home moving about the altar. Visitors to the church were sometimes not even aware that I was blind. One visitor, for example, asked about the symbolical meaning of the white staff which I carried. One of the members of the church had to explain to the visitor that I was blind and that it was not a shepherd's staff which I carried but the ordinary white cane of a blind person.

My fading eyesight also affected my other activities. At first I found that I could still mow the grass, because I could see a difference between the sheen of the cut grass and the grass not cut, but by the second year, I knew that I had to devise some other scheme. So I painted a number of white stakes and drove them into the edge of the lawn on one side of the yard at about twenty-foot intervals. I would then head for these stakes which I could dimly see across the lawn. Sometimes the neighborhood children would come over and say, "You missed a spot there," and with their help I managed to do a pretty good job. But after that second year, still other techniques had to be devised. One was to put the radio somewhere out ahead of me, mow toward it, and then mow parallel to the first mowing, always moving a little to the right of the radio, then a little farther to the right. In this way I was able to cut pretty good squares, and by moving the radio after a certain length of time and continuing the process, I was able to do the lawn all right. After a while, though, I just let the lawn grow a little longer. I could then feel just exactly how far I had gone with the mower. We had quite a piece of lawn in the front yard and also in the back, and this gave me plenty of exercise. In fact, I'm sure I got a lot more exercise out of mowing the lawn than anybody else could have.

The yard about our house became for me an increasingly important source of exercise, recreation, and soothing of the spirit. Since 1966, I had planted dwarf fruit trees, and now besides the original apples, plums, and pears, we had peaches, nectarines, and apricots. These required care, pruning, and spraying. At first the pruning was no great problem because I could still see the outline of the tree against the sky, but as the trees grew and my eyesight waned, I often had to rely on the advice of my neighbor, Bill Metcalf. With his help, even the hedges that enclosed two sides of the yard could be handled after a fashion. We simply determined that the hedge should be just the height of my breastbone, and would cut off everything that grew above that line.

Spraying the trees in spring was also a problem. First of all I had to be sure that I knew where the wind was blowing from, and second, I had to take a stance that would put me in proper relationship to the tree. When you have to do this by feeling for the tree, you can get a little bit out of line and every once in a while Bill Metcalf's voice would come across the yard and tell me that I was not spraying anything in particular and if I would like to spray the tree I should turn a few degrees this way or that.

Laying out a garden after the first year became a problem also. We managed however by taking a white plastic clothesline and outlining the edges of the garden with it, setting steel fence posts at corners. When it came to planting the rows, Clara and I devised a plan of setting stakes at about fifteen-inch intervals at either side of the garden and then connecting them with a piece of white plastic clothesline. At first this was visible to me, and it helped me very much in planting the rows. But even after I could no longer see the clothesline, it still served as a guide for my hands. I could plant the seed always to the right of the clothesline. Certain plants were easily distinguishable: tomatoes, broccoli, cabbage, and potatoes. Carrots were a problem because they send up such a fine feathery little shoot, but if one plants a few radish seeds along with the carrots, the radishes outline the row and the difficulty is taken care of. I think when I became completely blind, I got as much satisfaction out of feeling a garden grow as any sighted gardener gets out of seeing his grow.

In my garden there was a definite shift away from flowers to vegetables. The smell of an onion or the smell of a tomato plant became just as fragrant to me as the smell of the earliest flowers. I did keep on adding rose bushes from year to year and took care of them by what I called a system of "judicious neglect," fertilizing and pruning them blindly but managing to get some very lovely roses just the same.

My vacations were still spent at Lake James in northeastern Indiana where we had had a cottage in the family for some fifty years. I could still go fishing by myself because I knew the lake very well. At first, I could still see the outline of the shore, and as I drew near, could distinguish landmarks that told me when I was close to home. But as time went on, I had special reason to be grateful to cousin Wilfred, who continued to accept me as his fishing partner. I still knew the lake very well and could give him advice as to the directions in which we should travel, where we might anchor, how deep we should anchor, where we would find the edge of a sunken island, and so on. Thus we managed to continue our long association and pursue the blue gill with the same zest as before. Our conversation did not lag, and the stories and the reminiscences remained good.

Since I could no longer see a bobber, I had to fish with a free line, and this made it necessary to regain some childhood skills. Back in the days when I was very young and fished over the side of the boat, I could watch as the fish bit the hook, or at least feel it and so set the hook by feel. Now I had to do the same thing with the use of a pole. With a little practice it worked out very well. In fact, I got to the point where I would put two hooks about two feet apart on a line so that if the fish were down a little lower, I might catch them there; and if they were up a little higher, I might catch them there.

At Lake James I found another source of recreation too: I would take my tape recorder out to the road and tape the bird calls that I heard. Since at the start I could not identify any birds even when they came very close, I took more and more interest in the sounds they made. My sister had given me a set of bird-call records, and I was soon able to distinguish quite a range of birds, the Maryland yellow throat with his distinctive song as well as the oven bird, the catbird, the cardinal, the blue jay, the song sparrow, the red-winged blackbird, the brown thrasher, the wood thrush, the mourning dove, the towhee, the yellow-breasted chat, and many others. Unfortunately, I could not get these calls except against a background of noise from motorboats on the lake or cars on the highway. One morning I talked Clara into getting up early and driving me some ten miles to a place called Nevada Mills, where I was sure there were plenty of birds. There were, but I had forgotten that the Indiana toll road ran about a mile away from this particular location. So I had gotten away from the motor boats and one expressway only to run afoul again. Nevertheless, there are places where one can do such taping with a great deal of pleasure, and it is highly recommended for a blind person who cannot see birds but who can certainly enjoy the music that they make.

Swimming continued to be a pleasure, although it was fraught with its own problems. At first I could see the white boards on the pier and walk out without much trouble. The second year I could see the boards only with difficulty. One day someone laid a towel on the pier at an angle, and I carelessly did not realize that instead of following the pier I was following this towel. The first thing I knew I had stepped off the pier and fallen into the water. Fortunately, the boat which was usually moored there was in use and no harm was done. But a blind person always had to be on the lookout for things like this. My wife couldn't help but laugh, because it had been a saying in my family for some forty years that we were never really settled in at the lake until Bob fell into the water.

As my sight waned, I had to be a bit more careful when swimming. If I swam out to where the water was up to my shoulders, I could continue in almost any direction and not know where I was going. If I swam out into the middle of the lake, I did not know how long it would take me to get back to the shore—if I could tell which direction the shore was. I learned after a while to listen for certain noises. The people next door to us had a little cascade that ran from the front of their house to the lake. This made a splashing sound that I could distinguish unless it was a very, very stormy day. Of course, if it was a stormy day, I could hear the crash of the waves against the rocks along the shore. On the other side of our cottage a sailboat was moored. It had a line that went up to the top of the mast, and on that line was a metal ring which made clinking noises. So if I ever got out into the lake too far, I simply listened for the clank of that ring on the mast or the sound of the water trickling down from the cascade, and I could make my way back to my pier. Another problem was to be able to feel the pier without running into it. If there was a boat moored and some waves, I could hear them splash against the boat and that would tell me where the pier was. If there were no boats, I had to grope around.

Back home, St. John's congregation continued to take my problems in stride. In some situations, in fact, blindness was an advantage. In counseling, for example, some people seemed relieved of a fear that the pastor could scrutinize them and pass judgment on their face, their clothes, or anything of that kind. These people were more relaxed because they knew I would judge them only by what they said and that I could not detect some of the things which made them particularly ashamed or uneasy. The adult membership classes did not decline in numbers, but rather grew after I became blind. As stated the Bethel Bible series flourished tremendously, and it was most inspiring to see 250 and more people coming every Wednesday night. The congregation had never experienced anything like this before, and it was the beginning of a new spirit, a harbinger of better things to come. The study of the Bible had opened up God's revelation to these people in a way that was beneficial to them personally and to the work of the congregation as a whole.

At this time I looked about for new fields to conquer.

There were several directions in which we could go. Evangelism was standing still and needed some new impetus. The social ministry program had possibilities, and a new daughter congregation ought to be founded. This would take thinking and work. There was the continuing problem of reaching all the contacts that we had, following up on them, and neither I nor Pastor Brown had solved this problem by any means.

But it seemed to me that I should first equip myself better for working as a blind person in the situation in which God continued to leave me. Thinking about this reminded me that when I first became blind, a man from the social agency concerned with blind people had visited me. He was the area counselor and asked me if I wanted to pursue Braille or something of this kind and if I wanted to go away for further training. When he heard I had a system of drivers and readers and was able to continue my work, he thought that I probably would not need this sort of assistance, and did not press the matter further. Now the situation had changed a bit, and I had had some experience as a blind person working day by day in a congregation.

By the kindness of one of my members I had received records of the King James Version of the Bible and also a tape of the Today's English Version of the New Testament. This assisted me a great deal in the study of the Scriptures, in looking up texts, and in getting the meaning out of them. But it was a limited aid, and I looked about for some way in which I could do more independent reading and study of the Scriptures. From time to time I had wondered about Braille, and it began to seem to me that this would be an answer to some of my needs.

Beyond that, I needed better mobility. I walked about with a cane. I could take walks around the church, following the sidewalk and using an ordinary walking cane to tap away at the corners, but I had no desire to cross the street, nor did I have any confidence that I could get across safely. All I could do was walk about the church, enjoy the fresh air, and say hello to people now and then. I was pretty well limited to the block on which the church sat. Even in my home area I could only walk up and down the street.

Finally I consulted with a young woman from the Social Services Bureau who was now area counselor for the blind. She told me that she thought that the institution that would serve me best was the Rehabilitation Center for the Blind in Kalamazoo. This was a state institution which a blind person could attend without cost. I would be obligated for my travel expenses, but room, board, tuition—all of these things were taken care of. In addition, a wide program of study was offered, the chief idea being to enable young people just graduated from high school to find an occupation in which they could support themselves and to help older people, who had perhaps dropped active work, to find some way in which they still could become gainfully employed.

The Center at Kalamazoo represented a centralization of various efforts which had been carried out in different parts of the state. It was felt that with one faculty, one unified program, the blind could be helped in a better and more efficient way. The local school districts generally took care of the education of children from the lower grades through high school, and special education was carried out in most every school district by law. Though there was still a school for the blind at Lansing, the time was coming when the local school districts would be likely to take over the burden, and blind young people would learn to get along with sighted young people instead of being with other blind people in a special school. Young people who graduated from the school at Lansing generally had some skills—musical skills, typing skills, and sometimes some skill at woodworking or something of this sort, but they were by no means ready to step into a regular job, and the Rehabilitation Center was to help them in this.

There was always danger that a blind person, finding

himself so dependent, will become completely dependent and look for the easy way out. This could mean simply accepting a blind pension and living as well as possible on that pension. But the Rehabilitation Center for the Blind wanted to help blind people find places in certain other fields which were opening up for them. Piano tuning had long been a field for some of the young men, and now the field of servicing vending machines in public buildings, government buildings, was open. The field of medical transcription was also opening up. Doctors were now making their reports on tapes, and a blind person could transcribe these tapes as well an anyone else. So there were opportunities, and the large number of counselors at the Rehabilitation Center for the Blind were as anxious to help young people find work as were the area counselors throughout the state.

I went into this rather blindly, thinking only of Braille and mobility, not knowing the wide spread of the courses that were offered at the Rehabilitation Center, but after some negotiations with the area counselor and directly with the authorities in Kalamazoo, I received word that I would be admitted to the school in the early part of December 1972. The elders of the congregation and the church council gave their wholehearted approval to the project, telling me to take as much time as I needed, no matter how long I would have to be away from the congregation. And so one fine day in December, with the usual assistance of my faithful drivers, I headed for Kalamazoo and a most enlightening period in my life. Personally, I looked upon it as a counterattack—a counterattack against blindness, against dependency, against my handicapped status—and I hoped for great things from this experience.

Chapter 5
New Tools and Weapons

So it came to pass in early December 1972 that the ever-ready transportation service of St. John's church brought Clara and me to the Rehabilitation Center for the Blind and Physically Handicapped at Kalamazoo, which lay on a main north-south street near Western Michigan University and right across the street from an institution for the mentally retarded. The Rehab Center was located in a building about three years old, built roughly in the shape of a capital "G," the base of the "G" fronting along the main street. It included offices, counselors' rooms, a small auditorium where hearing tests were given, classrooms, a gymnasium, and an all-purpose auditorium. A special entrance to the building led to the kitchen and served as the main entrance for students, who were admitted by ringing a bell that alerted the kitchen staff. There was also a library and a general purpose game room with a billiard table, other games that the blind and partly sighted can play, a piano, and a television set. A lounge contained tables, comfortable chairs and couches, another television set, and some vending machines for snacks and drinks. A two-story section of the building included the men's dormitory, nurse's office, laundry, and the girl's dormitory (or "never-never land"). A courtyard in the open space of the "G" could be reached from a number of directions, and a tiny chapel was used for Bible class and the Abacus class.

Behind the building was a large area about the size of several football fields. Here a bicycle track of blacktop followed the somewhat rolling contour of the land. Blind people could ride on this track if they didn't go too fast and remembered some of the main features of the track. Since my stay at the Center was during the winter and early spring months, not much bicycling was done, but the pathway was nevertheless used for taking walks and for getting a bit of fresh air.

My arrival, while expected, was inopportune, because Mrs. Jacobs, who was in charge of the placement of new arrivals, had suffered an injury. The new person, who was to be my counselor, had not yet arrived, and so the burden of acquainting me with the grounds fell upon Robert Hall, a genial person who was in charge of Mobility. He pointed out the main features of the building and gave me little tips such as the information that door handles for outside doors were rough, while those for inside doors were smooth. He pointed out other areas, then took me upstairs to Room 2 in the men's dormitory. The numbers were on the doors in large, raised letters. Mine turned out to be a single room, though I shared a bath with Room 1. The room was not exactly Spartan in its simplicity, but was simple nevertheless. A window across from the door could act as a guide for a person with some light perception. To the right was a closet, a built-in bureau, and a place to keep a suitcase. Continuing along the right wall I came to a lounge chair, and, in the far right corner, a small desk with a drawer and a chair. The bed paralleled the window, and on the left-hand side of the room stood a little nightstand, then a washstand which protruded into the room. Its position was probably carefully planned, but it presented some sharp surfaces that left dents on your head if you were not careful. A bright light in this little cubicle also served to guide persons with light perception. Next came the door to the bathroom, which consisted of a tub, a shower, and a toilet. And that was it.

There were about 35 students at this time, and this remained average during the time I was there, though the dormitories would hold forty to fifty people. Signs everywhere indicated that this was an institution for the blind. All the doors were inscribed with the official title of the room in Braille. The cards in the game room were Braille cards, and the first thing I received from the hands of Mr. Hall himself was a cane, the official cane used by the Rehabilitation Center for the Blind and advocated by the School at Western Michigan University. It is called a "long cane," and is made of aluminum with a cork handle grip and a nylon tip which is replaceable. This nylon tip becomes quite sharp from scraping constantly across cement sidewalks, and one must be careful when walking in company with women not to swing the cane across the lady's leg for fear of doing violence to her hose. The cane comes up to the center of the breastbone, just about at the solar plexis, and is used for reaching out and exploring. The Mobility Department helps blind persons develop a technique for the use of this cane, which enables them to travel safely in most circumstances.

Everybody was on a first-name basis at the Center. The staff called the students by their first names, and on almost all occasions the students responded by calling the teachers by their first names. This was also true of the kitchen staff and the people who kept up the building. During the course of that first afternoon, Bob Hall eventually turned me over to a young man by the name of Bill, who was partly sighted, and he took me in hand in a very nice way. The experience of meeting so many blind people at one time was an overwhelming one for me. I had hardly ever met a blind person. I had found out myself what the problems were, but to meet some 35 blind people, one after the other, was quite an experience.

Initiation began at supper time. I found out that you hung your cane, which had identification in Braille on it, on a rack. Fortunately, I had memorized the Braille alphabet before coming to the school, and so I could distinguish the markings on my cane. Usually there were a person's initials, but since mine were similar to many others, they put my nickname, Bob, on my cane. It was very easy to get confused especially when you were a tyro at Braille. The very first day one of the girls gave me some cord to hang on my cane and distinguish it. "Because," she said, "unless you know Braille pretty well, you'll be getting the wrong cane or not be able to find your cane at all." I was grateful for that hint, and the cord lasted until I was home and picked up a little plastic cross to fasten to the cane.

When I left the cafeteria line, I felt rather on my own, but I soon found that many people were anxious to meet a new student, even if he was a super-annuated old man. They hadn't discovered this yet, let alone that he was a minister, and they called and invited me to come over and sit with them.

Conversation began with someone saying, "Hi, are you the new person here?"

"Yes, I am the new person," I replied.

"What's your name?"

"Robert Weller."

"But what do you call yourself?"

I hesitated. Everybody had called me Butch, but I thought I'd compromise with Bob. Everybody laughed, because there were no less than six Bobs on the faculty, and so it was a little confusing. The others told me their names and where they came from, and we were friends right from the start, because the blind person is always seeking closer relationships with people. In fact, relationships at the Center were so close that we had two weddings during the time that I was there, and most all of the boys and girls were paired off in one way or another.

The balance between the staff and the student body at the Center was held at almost a one-to-one ratio. In Mobility we always worked on a one-to-one basis. In the Braille class there would be two, occasionally three people, with a teacher at any one time. In Occupational Therapy, Woodworking, and Techniques of Daily Living, there would seldom be more than two or three people in each class.

Students were at the Center for various purposes. Some

wanted to prepare themselves for a definite occupation, some wanted to go on to college, some wanted to improve their Braille, and some wanted to take up Mobility for the first time. A few of the older ones were going blind, and wanted to prepare for that day before it came. There was one old lady who wanted to learn enough Braille so she could make labels to put on the fruit and vegetables that she canned. She lived alone and identifying what she was opening had been a constant problem to her. One woman wanted to learn just enough Mobility so she could bring in the mail, do other little chores of this kind, and so enrich her life a little. Many took great interest in things like Occupational Therapy and hand work of various kinds.

That first evening in the cafeteria I came to feel very much at home. I was seated at a table with both young girls and fellows, and there was a lot of joking and laughing. One vivacious girl seemed to be the center of all this and I found out that her name was Sonja. When she discovered that I was a Lutheran minister, she said, "You don't happen to be of the Missouri Synod, do you?"

I said, "Yes," and she said, "I come from Pastor Unger's church in Detroit."

I said, "I know Pastor Unger and his wife and their children very well," and found out that Sonja lived next door to the Ungers. So we had many things to talk about and she introduced me to others. That night as I lay down in my own room for the first time, I assessed the situation and realized that I had had no idea of what I was getting into when I first made my plans. I had simply decided to gain a knowledge of Braille and mobility, and now I saw that I would be able to learn these things and many others against a very sociable and comfortable background.

At this time my own eyesight had reached the point where I had only light vision out of the corner of my left eye. I could tell where the windows were in a room, and if I were outside, I could generally locate the sun, but sometimes I did that by the warmth of its rays more than by the concentration of light. Once in a while I could see a flash of color. One day one of the girls was standing next to me, and I thought I saw an area of pink off to my left shoulder. When I asked the girl what color dress she was wearing, she said, "I'm wearing a very bright pink dress."

I said, "I can see that, and I thought that's what you would be wearing."

She exclaimed over this, because a blind person always thinks it's wonderful if another blind person can see anything at all.

I didn't realize until I talked with another girl that a person who has always been blind has no concept of color at all.

"I have no conception of any color at all," she said. "They tell me that what I see is black and gray, but I have never seen anything else. Even in my dreams, I see nothing but what I have seen when I am awake.

She said she was acquainted with spheres, squares, and other objects from feeling them with her hands, and so she dreamed about them as symbolical shapes. Of course, her dreams could be filled with fear and joy, but there were no clear pictures of any kind.

In spite of the fact that some of the girls and boys had no concept of color at all, they sewed little washable metal tags onto their shirts and other clothing so they would put on things that matched. A Braille character on the tags tells the color of the article.

It means nothing to the person who is blind that our flag is red, white, and blue. You might just as well tell him that it is one, two and three. But at this time, my own vision had reached a stage where I had red, white, and blue phases, perhaps in preparation for the Bicentennial of the country. In my white phases I couldn't see a thing, but in any direction that I looked, everything seemed to be lit up with a brilliant white light. The blue phase suddenly, without any warning, produced an aquamarine flow of color into my whole field of vision—such field of vision as a blind person has. Wherever I looked, instead of seeing the usual gray, I saw a very pretty aquamarine. On still

66

other occasions, a dull rose-pink would flow through my field of vision. These three colors continued to come to me from time to time and still surge into my consciousness. Whether they have a physical cause or are just moods, I have no idea, but I often wonder if people who have been blind all their lives experience them too and just don't recognize them as colors.

Personally, I'm very grateful for the dreams I have. They are some of the happiest hours of my life. I dream of fields whose green is beyond reality, and the same vividness of color holds true for my flowers and my birds. It is as if my subconscious mind is trying to make up for the fact that I don't see anything at all now.

People who are born blind have a certain sense which is very valuable to them and generally does not come to people who are blind later in life. One of the girls would walk down the street with me and say, "I hear a telephone pole," or "I hear a lamp post," or "I hear a car." And she would reach over with her cane and tap the car or the telephone pole or the lamp post. I was able to check her out on the lamp post, because I could look up and see the light at the top out of the corner of my eye. She was never wrong. I think that this is something that a blind person develops as a very young child, something that they unconsciously develop, an ability to hear either the echo of a sound or even the change in air pressure as they approach something. When this girl was in doubt about something, she would stamp her feet. If the echo did not come back to her strongly enough, she would stamp her feet again in order to make a stronger echo. She could go down a corridor and tell which of the doors were open simply by the response she received. This is a very useful thing, and I saw blind people moving around tables in the cafeteria without running into anything. I blundered into things continually. Once in a while, I feel as if I am developing this sense when I stop just short of bumping into a wall or something like that, but this generally happens in the house where I'm aware of the location of things. Outside I sometimes run smack into something at full tilt, which is not only embarrassing but very painful.

I also found that some people express strange attitudes toward their vision. Occasionally I would hear two blind people talking together, and one would say, "Remember Joe?"

"Yeah."

"Well, he got his sight back, and he said he didn't like it."

"Yeah, I don't think I'd like it either."

Now it's hard to assess such a statement, and I wonder if perhaps when such a person does receive his sight, he is overwhelmed by the responsibility that falls upon him. He can no longer be dependent. He can see, and so he has to take upon himself all sorts of chores and duties and responsibilities that he didn't have to take before. His security is shaken. He has to be more independent, and perhaps it is this he does not like. I cannot imagine not being happy at being able to see again, but I can see that my life would change radically. I'd have to drive for myself; I'd have to read for myself; I'd have to change a lot of things, and some of them would be chores.

I find that all kinds of odd things happen to me because I am blind. Some time ago, some friends brought me home from the church, pulled up in the driveway and let me off. I assured them I could find my way into the house but noticed that I could still hear the motor of their car running outside in the driveway. I closed the door and still could hear the car. Finally, I heard them drive away. The next day I happened to run across one of them, and asked if they had had any trouble in the driveway.

My friend laughed and said, "No, we were just waiting for you to turn on the light so that we could see that you were all right."

I laughed too and said, "I'm sorry. I just walk into the house and never think of turning on the light."

At the Center you are carefully trained to put your hand upon a chair before you sit down lest you sit down upon a pie or somebody's hat, or even a lady's lap. I have never failed to sit down comfortably except on the one instance in my own office. I have two identical chairs, both with arm rests. Normally I sit down without any difficulty, but one day I was thinking about something else, and put my right arm on the left arm rest of one chair and my left arm on the right arm rest of the other chair. Then I neatly sat down between them.

But when you come into people's homes for the first time, they are very solicitous about guiding you safely to a chair. They will say, "Just a little bit to your right." But since they are facing you, they really mean to the left. And they will say, "Now if you will just come this way," when they really mean that they want you to back up. Usually I can reach around with my cane, make contact with a chair, and find my own way to it better than I can follow the directions of an inexperienced person. People are also always concerned about my getting safely down their front steps. If I have a cane, there is no danger and they don't need to worry. But they do anyway, and they want to be helpful. Just as I am carefully stepping off the first step, they grab my arm and lift me up, which throws me off balance and is likely to bring both of us tumbling down the steps. It would be all right if they offered me their arm, but when they take mine and lift me up, they are doing me a disservice.

Sometimes people ask whether one's other faculties don't become more acute when one loses one's sight. Doesn't one's hearing, touch, and smell all become sharper, more adequate? I don't think this is the case. I think they remain as sharp as they ever were, but we make better use of them now. Hearing is a sense that I make much more use of than I ever did before. When I go out in the yard, I always listen for sounds about the neighborhood. If somebody is mowing the lawn, then I remember that it is the person to the north of me, and that gives me a point of reference. If I do get lost in the yard, I stop and listen for the sound of traffic on a nearby main street, and this immediately gets me properly oriented again.

But back to the Center. My education began at 8 o'clock on Tuesday morning. I had been given a schedule which I could not read, but one of the girls told me where I was to go. Mobility came first, and Bob Hall introduced me to the intricacies of the proper way to tap with a cane. It was to be swung from side to side, describing an arc that begins one inch to the outside of the left shoulder and ends up one inch to the right of the right shoulder. In this manner, the cane is always exploring the area where the next footstep will fall, and when the technique is properly carried out, it will be safe for the blind person to put his foot down in the place that has been explored by the cane. There will not be a bicycle in the way or a pair of roller skates or a trench of a curb. It is difficult sometimes to get into the rhythm of this, and my first days were spent in a great deal of practice.

The next most important course for me was Braille. Suzanne Johnson, the teacher, was herself blind and could perform such clever feats as walking around the room with a Braille book held against her hip, reading as she walked. I learned that everything is centered around the Braille cell, a group of six dots like those on a die or domino. These dots are numbered, the left-hand side 1, 2, 3, the right-hand side 4, 5, 6. I learned to use a slate made up of four lines of twenty-eight braille cells and a stylus for punching out dots. Since you want to feel the dots on the opposite side of the paper after you have finished, you must always make the letters in reverse order, from right to left, so that they will appear correctly when you turn the paper over. This takes a bit of doing, and is especially confusing because with the Braille typewriter, you don't have to reverse things. I started with just a few letters, learned these, then began putting them together into small words. My real problem was lack of sensitivity in my fingers. At one time Suzanne said, "I don't know if it is really worthwhile for you to continue, because you often say that you can't feel a certain letter." But I was stubborn and determined, and either practice paid off or some sensitivity returned to my fingers, because I eventually got to the point where I could read Braille well enough for my purposes.

Other courses included one that I called "Old Testament," since it was abbreviated "OT." OT actually stood for Occupational Therapy and covered all kinds of things. Various tests were given at the beginning of the class, sensitivity tests, recognition tests, etc. The teacher was a young woman called Pam. At first I thought of her as a blond flibbertigibbet, but I found out after a while that she was brunette and very dedicated to her tasks.

Another course was Techniques of Daily Living, abbreviated TDL. Here we did everything from dusting and making beds to cooking, and I was happy to be told on one occasion that I had a very good dusting technique, a good sweep that efficiently covered the area I was trying to dust. High praise!

Finally, there was a course called Aural and Oral Techniques. This involved tape recorders and other kinds of electronic equipment, about which a great deal of information was available. The director of this class was a fine Christian person called Bob Lovett, who made it possible for people to go to church and provided transportation if necessary. He himself had spent considerable time in Germany, and his wife had come from Germany. He had a pretty good command of the German language, and when he found out that I could speak German, we generally exchanged a few German greetings.

In a few days, I met the woman who was to be my counselor, Mrs. Florence McCulley. It turned out that I had known members of her family in Rogers City. She was a most considerate and sympathetic person, who went out of her way to assist me in adjusting to life at the Center. In my case, there weren't too many personal problems that she had to relate to, so often our counseling was a matter of discussing various religious, philosophical, and literary issues, which was most pleasant.

As soon as I had settled into the routine of the Center, I began to plan how I might occasionally go back to Midland and do at least a share of the work in the congregation. I knew that it was a policy of the Center to ask new students to stay for at least a month before they went home, but in my case they shaved this requirement. I stayed for the first three Sundays and then went home for the Christmas holidays and returned after the New Year. My counselor and I tentatively agreed that I could operate in this way, going home now and then for a whole week, or ten days, so that I might keep up with my work. Practically no one else at the Center was in this situation with a job in which they were actively engaged and a certain work load with which they had to keep up. It finally worked out so that each month I was at the Center for eighteen days and in Midland for about twelve days. While I was at the Center, I worked on sermons for the weekends that I would be home, and while I was at home in Midland, I worked on lessons in Braille that my instructor had provided.

As Christmas approached, the same feelings arose in the hearts of the blind people as arise in the hearts of people everywhere before Christmas. They wanted their own Christmas tree, and they didn't want it set up in the main lobby where officialdom held sway. They wanted it in their own lounge and this was arranged. Soon the fragrance of the tree began to permeate the lounge. The OT department got people working on Christmas tree ornaments, and soon everybody was hanging the ornament that he or she had fashioned. Each person came up to finger the various ornaments and to smell the tree, and the halls began to ring with the sound of Christmas carols.

One of the girls, Alberta, told me how she had gone out the preceding Christmas at home and foraged in the yard for anything she could find that smelled nice. She found pieces of evergreen, dried weeds, and dried flowers and arranged them all in what she thought was a lovely, fine smelling bouquet in a vase in her room. But when her mother saw it, she said, "That looks terrible. Throw it out." So regretfully Alberta threw away what to her had been something fine because it smelled so nice, and all because of the lack of sympathy of a sighted person for an unsighted person. One of the nicest gifts I have received was a carved carabao from the Philippines, where my daughter and her husband were spending some years in the Peace Corps. It was pleasant for me to finger the wooden image and see exactly what a carabao is like, and it was also nice to feel the smoothness of the polished wood, the grain, and even the muscles that the craftsman had given to the beast.

Plans were made for a Christmas party several days before the students would go home, and everybody worked on some little thing to contribute, a song, a poem, or something else to enliven the proceedings. I had an idea for a way in which I could make some of the members of St. John's more aware of blind people. We had a number of students from the church attending Western Michigan University, and one day I got in touch with three of the girls and invited them to go out on a little supper party with me and one of the girls from the Rehab Center. For the occasion I chose Sonja, because she would be going home for good in a short time. The girls knew the town, and agreed to come in a taxi and pick us up. We had a pretty good supper, and I was delighted to see how Sonja responded to this opportunity to let the younger girls know what life was like at the Center. Sonja was in her early thirties, with three children, and so she had special difficulties and problems, but she was a lively person and impressed the girls very much.

At the end of the meal, everyone else chose modest desserts, but I opted for something with ice cream, chocolate cake and syrup, whipped cream, and a cherry. I had no idea what it would look like when it came. The girls oh'd and ah'd, but before they could warn me that the thing stood some fifteen inches high, I grabbed a spoon and leaned down, pushing my face, nose, and a few other parts of my anatomy into the pile of whipped cream. This was the greatest joke of the evening, and put an end to any dignity that I might have preserved.

On the Thursday evening before we were to go home for Christmas, Jan Luertsema wanted to do something in the way of saying farewell to Sonja, her roommate, and I suggested that I would be glad to be the host again for a little dinner for the three of us. Since they also wanted to go shopping for some jingle bells, we could combine the shopping tour with this little farewell party. Jan had considerable vision, so she was most helpful in getting us on the right bus and off at the right stop.

As we ate, we joked, especially about putting the Elmer's Glue in one of Jan's eyes that tended to wander. This sort of joke may seem crude to sighted persons, but I think that the blind learn to handle their handicaps by speaking of them in such a way. It's not unusual for one blind person, walking down the corridor at the Center, to say to another blind person who has bumped into the water fountain, "What's the matter, stupid? Are you blind?" This reaction is, I think, somewhat explained by a little quotation from Thomas Moore at the beginning of C. S. Lewis' *The Screw Tape Letters:* "The devil, that proud spirit, cannot stand to be mocked." I think this is the way blind people often handle their handicaps and the trials and irritations which the devil places in their way. They laugh at them, and this is probably best.

After dinner, Sonja, Jan, and I began our quest for the jingle bells. We were in the midst of a shopping center, so we went first to a ten-cent store area, or as close as you can come to a ten-cent store in these days of inflation, but they had no jingle bells, and suggested another area which sold Christmas decorations. With Jan's help, we made our way to that area, but they had no jingle bells either. They suggested a third area and we went over there. No jingle bells. Finally, in desperation, we began asking shoppers where we might find our bells. Some kind person said, "If you will go to Frank's." Frank's is a chain nursery that sells seasonal decorations of all kinds. So we set out in search of Frank's. We were told that it was not in the mall proper but across a parking lot. One poor set of directions led us only to a dark street and after being misguided a second time, we returned to the mall and went up to a kindly old lady standing in a booth. Again we explained that we were looking for Frank's Nursery and asked if she could direct us. She said she certainly could.

"You go out that door to your right and there is the parking lot. You make your way across that parking lot, and you will come to a very, very bright light. That marks Frank's. Find the entrance there, and they can direct you to what you want."

We thanked her profusely, but just as we were about to leave she added, "Oh, you know that parking lot is just terrible. There are hills of ice and snow. It would be much better if you wouldn't walk. Doesn't any of you drive?"

We stood there, leaning on our white canes and tried not to laugh. We said, "No, none of us drives," and hurried out the side door where we could enjoy the joke in private, because nothing seemed more humorous and ridiculous to us than the question, "Doesn't any of you drive?"

As we made our way across the parking lot, we stopped at intervals and inquired of one another. "Didn't you bring your driver's license? Why didn't you bring your car? Doesn't any of you drive?" And we would go off again into gales of laughter. This kept up our party spirit. It was a good thing because ours was indeed a perilous journey. Jan went first; I took her hand; and Sonja was the tail of the kite, whipping from right to left. I could not see what was going on; I could only follow Jan and found myself sliding up the sides of snow hills and then down icy little inclines, holding on to Sonja as best I could. But the strength of our laughter carried us across that lot and at last we reached Frank's, the Mecca where we found our jingle bells!

Shortly before Christmas, a new girl, called Carol, came in. She had suffered her first diabetic hemorrhage, a severe one, and had been almost completely blind for several days. This frightened her, and when she found out what the prognosis might be for the future, she determined to come to the Center and begin to take as much training as she could against the day when she might lose her sight completely. At first she was quite nervous about the situation, but she was kindly received by the young people at the Center, had an engaging personality, and turned out to be very helpful to us, because her vision began to return. Carol was our guide on another hilarious shopping expedition which involved a partly sighted boy named Bill S. who had to exchange a blouse which was to be a Christmas present for his girl friend. Alberta also wanted to buy a blouse, so the four of us headed downtown. Bill first returned his blouse, and there Alberta began her shopping. Bill and Carol tried to describe to her the colors in the blouses she was picking, and she tried to decide whether she liked the "feel" of the material or not. We all followed Alberta around wherever she went, and, as sometimes happens, forgot that just because we couldn't see other people didn't mean they couldn't see us. All of a sudden a salesgirl came over and said, "I'll have to ask you to leave. This is the women's dressing room."

Bill and I sidled out shamefacedly and went elsewhere to wait for Alberta to make her decision. In a few minutes she too came out, and we went over to a counter to pay for the blouse. While she was completing her transaction, I stood beside the counter and aimlessly groped around to see what was on the counter. I encountered something I couldn't identify and kept sliding my hand up a smooth surface until Carol came over and laughingly said, "You ought to be ashamed of yourself."

I said, "What's the matter?"

"You are being very disrespectful to a young lady."

"To a young lady?"

"What you have your hand on is a mannequin," she informed me, "and the mannequin has on only a very brief pair of panties. You seem intent on removing those panties."

To cover my embarrassment, I said to the salesgirl, "What is the sale price on these mannequins?"

She stuttered for a moment, and she said, "Well-l-l, I-I-I don't think they are on sale."

I retreated after this, and in a short time we were on our way home.

At last our Christmas party was held, and the girls danced around with the hard-won jingle bells sewed to their skirts. There was group singing, solos, little dialogs, other kinds of entertainment, and refreshments. Everybody said, "Happy Christmas," and then it was time to go home.

Christmas at home was the same glorious festival it always was. I was overwhelmed with the realization that in spite of my blindness, I could still serve in my church. I could tell my people about Christmas. I could tell them that the birth of Jesus Christ showed the inexpressible love of God for each and every one of us and His desire to have all men to be saved and come to the knowledge of the truth.

At the same time I felt that there was a ministry for me at the Center too. Shortly before I came home for Christmas one of the girls had asked if she could talk to me. The question which she posed was this: "Do you think that parents are ashamed of their child who is blind?" I pondered this for a moment, then asked her a few questions. I learned that she was one of several children. The others could work and earn good wages, but she worked in a sheltered workshop and her income was necessarily small. The others made good grades in school, their parents could be proud of them and praise them. But she had the feeling that her parents were simply ashamed of her.

I told her that I did not think this was the case at all. I said that I felt parents loved a blind child more than they loved their sighted children, even if they could not praise the blind child for any accomplishments. If parents sometimes seemed to act strangely toward a blind child, it was because they themselves felt guilty. In their hearts they never quite knew whether their child's blindness was due to some fault on their part. They feared that somehow they had failed their child. At other times, as parents often neglect to do, they just didn't express their love as richly as they should. I think the girl was somewhat comforted by this. We never spoke of it again, but we were always very good friends.

So the year 1973 began, and I was full of Christmas joy and hopes for the New Year. I discussed Braille with my teacher and told her that my goal was to be finished by Easter, because I wanted to be back home and in full service again in the congregation by then. We agreed that we would work toward this goal as diligently as we could. So with all of these happy thoughts, and, above all things, trusting that God had purposes to fulfill, I entered the new year.

Chapter 6
Marking Time—
Gathering Strength

During the first four months of 1973, I lost myself in my studies and my ministry at the Rehab Center and so kept from worrying about what might and should be happening at St. John's. Sonja had given me the magic telephone number for transportation on Sundays and other occasions to Zion Lutheran Church. Calling this number never failed, and I appreciated very much both the transportation and the services. In spite of the people's kindness, however, I did see another example of the shyness sighted persons have toward the blind. The people who transported me would let me off in the narthex of the church while they parked the car. Sometimes I stood for ten minutes waiting for them to return, and never was I approached by any member of the congregation, except on one occasion by somebody I had met before.

The weather in January kept us inside the Center most of the time, and so we worked at Brailling out rooms. We would be put inside a room, such as the game room, and told to take an inventory of what was in the room by going around the walls either clockwise or counterclockwise. We would first pass along the wall and locate pictures, light switches, alarm bells, thermostats, windows, doors, bookshelves, and any pieces of furniture that were so closely attached to the wall that we couldn't get behind them. After a complete circuit of the room, we would repeat our findings to Bob Hall. Then we walked straight across the room, to find out what stood in the way—tables, chairs, pool table, etc. Next we moved at a 45° angle in each direction. By that time, we had pretty well canvassed the room and knew what was in it and what we would meet up with in any direction. This technique was to be used for getting acquainted with any room in which we were going to spend some length of time. Whenever I am to preach at a church or speak at a hall, I like to Braille out the room first. It not only gives me confidence, but also enables me to project my voice in the proper directions, and thus maintain as much audience contact and even eye contact as a blind person can manage.

Sometimes we went into the lounge, and Bob would drop coins and let them roll. We were to try to listen to the course of the coin and see how close we could come to its stopping point and pick it up. I found this rather fascinating and learned all sorts of things about the sizes of coins and their idiosyncracies as they rolled.

We also spent some hours in the multipurpose room practicing our cane technique up and down the room and also going in a straight line from one side of the room to the other. This is an important technique for safely crossing streets from curb to curb, and we found that the better we mastered the careful arcing of the cane, the more likely we were to make a straight path across the room.

Bob also took me and other students over to the buildings at Western Michigan University. Our purpose was to go into one of the buildings, determine which was north so that we could always keep some sort of orientation as we moved around, and learn to find our way through the buildings. We were given certain problems to solve, such as reaching a certain room by listening to and carefully following directions. Once Bob asked me to find a commons room on the third floor. My clue would be a drinking fountain along the wall. When I approached the room from the right, I would come in contact with this drinking fountain and know that I was only a few feet from the door. Well, I carried out the instructions and came to the place where the drinking fountain should be. I even came to a door which seemed to be the one I was looking for, because I could hear people sitting around at tables, chairs scraping, and glasses clinking. But I had not found my clue, the drinking fountain. So I went back and retraced my steps. When Bob said "drinking fountain," I'd pictured one of those that's operated electrically and stands away from the wall, or else a pedestal type. This one, it seems, was completely recessed. When I passed the place in question the first time, I managed to slide my hand just over the top of it, and when I returned I slid my hand just under it. So I wandered off somewhere else and made a general botch of the whole problem, although I had had the solution almost under my fingers.

A variation of this business of going over to the University was to go out to one of the shopping malls. Bob would bring me to the door and give me instructions for finding a certain shop within the mall. I would then try to follow his directions and locate the proper place by some clue he had given me. Sometimes his clues turned out to be very elusive. Once he told me that I would recognize a certain place by the aroma of roasting nuts that came from it. Well, I followed the directions, but walked directly past the store because on that particular day they weren't doing any roasting. Bob trailed me and admitted that his clue wasn't valid that day.

As the weather changed in February and March, so did our work in Mobility. One day I received a tape from Bob. "Memorize this," he said. It was a description of a neighborhood about five blocks by eight blocks, and the tape told what streets came in what order, what direction they ran, what the cross streets were, and how they ran from block to block. By studying this tape, I eventually got a complete picture of that area, and was supposed to be able to find my way to any place in it. Now I was to practice my cane technique so that I actually could make the street crossings, follow the streets, beware of dead ends, and learn what to do when a sidewalk suddenly stopped and I had to go out in the street and follow the curb for a while.

At first I practiced simply following a sidewalk, avoiding going up or down a driveway, learning the slight slant that indicated something that led to the street, learning to recognize when I had gotten out to the street by the crown that usually exists in the center of the street. I also practiced crossing intersections in a straight line so I would reach the proper section of the sidewalk on the other side. All of this I did over and over again until the arcing of the came became automatic.

When I began to work in this area, there was still considerable snow and ice on some of the sidewalks, which involved me in several scrapes.

Once I came to an icy section that was quite slippery. I slithered this way and that and was relieved when finally I felt a piece of bare concrete beneath my cane. I did not notice that there was a slant to this concrete and since my cane continued to find something hard, I tapped merrily on my way, also oblivious of other clues that I would notice after more experience. I increased my pace, and then, all of a sudden, my cane crashed into something and I found myself inside a building. I felt around, came across a bicycle, and realized that I was in somebody's garage. I could not imagine just what I had done, but again knew that if I retraced my steps I should go down the driveway and come to the sidewalk. So I tapped down the driveway, found a sidewalk, turned right, and continued on my way. After a few steps, though, Bob Hall stopped me and said, "Where do you think you're headed?"

And I said, "I'm going the way I am supposed to go."

"Listen for the traffic," he said.

I listened and the traffic was on the wrong side of me. I had left the sidewalk, gone completely across the street, up a driveway, and then into a garage. Bob clucked his tongue, and then we went on to conquer new fields.

The weather finally cleared, and I got to the point where I was doing a lot of traveling downtown, practicing crossings where there were traffic lights. Crossing some of the large downtown streets where there are six lanes of traffic one way is somewhat of a thrilling experience. Approaching such a corner requires considerable attention to the sounds that one hears. You hear traffic going by in two directions, and you must locate the direction in which the traffic is going and also which traffic is halted and which is moving. Then you must find your curb and get a firm position on it so that you will start out at right angles to the street. Next you notice when the traffic crossing in front of you comes to a halt. You tense yourself to take off the moment you hear the roar of the traffic that is parallel to your path. The moment it starts, you start. In fact, if you can get the jump on it, so much the better. These drivers are supposed to see your cane, and if they are going to make a turn, they are responsible to see that they don't hit you. This, however, is very little comfort when you hear the roaring of engines, especially trucks or some heavy equipment, and you wonder just what's going to happen when you step off the curb. You are very much concerned about shifting your course so as not to go out into the traffic which you want to parallel, and you tend to veer toward the traffic that is waiting. Every once in a while you will run into the radiator of a car, or your cane will make contact with a tire or a fender. But there is a sort of unique exaltation and excitement in stepping out with the traffic and, well, wondering.

One new development, however, is becoming quite a problem for blind persons. It seems that some cities, states, and even the federal government have ordinances stating that all street crossings should consist of a ramp rather than a curb. A blind person is likely to walk right down a ramp and out into the traffic unless he is very much aware of every sound that comes to him. I hope that the federal government also makes some regulation requiring a roughened area or small ridge by the crossing. This will not hinder a bicycle or a wheelchair, but will warn the blind person that he is coming to the street.

All kinds of complications could occur on a mission. One day I was to go to a bank. I chose the wrong entrance and went into some kind of a loan department on the side, but somebody told me, "I'll take you to the proper part." I made the mistake of letting the person take me by the arm instead of asking to let me take him by the arm, and so I got scolded for that later. The next part of my assignment was to go into another building, find the elevator, and go up to the third floor to a certain office. It's a little difficult to take an elevator, and you have to find somebody to let you know when you get to the third floor, but I had no difficulty finding the building. I walked into the front door and heard the sound of an elevator, so I walked straight ahead until I came to a dead end. As I wondered which way I should turn now, a voice said to me. "Do you want to go up on the elevator, sir?" Apparently I had by accident walked directly into the elevator. The people on the elevator were apparently just as relieved to see that I wanted to go up with them as I was relieved to find out that they were people waiting in the elevator. We got up to the third floor and after I made the proper left-hand turn and counted the number of doors, I came to an office where Bob was making one of his payments. He often combined business with business.

Toward the end of the training we had to do some rather difficult things, such as making our own telephone calls to the bus company and finding out just precisely what time a bus left, what time we could make a connection at a certain corner, and where the bus we wanted to make connections with would be waiting. I went through this rigmarole one afternoon, and the next morning started out about eight o'clock, catching the bus in front of the Center and going downtown. I got off at the proper corner and then prepared to square off for a crossing of six lanes of traffic to catch my bus which was to be across the street. Now across the street, unfortunately, is a misleading term. It can be directly across the street if this is a street with two-way traffic, but this was a street with only one-way traffic, and so the bus was waiting on the side street. I was thinking that across the street meant on the other side of the same street that I was now going to cross and I made the following blunder.

According to Bob, I started out with a perfect sense of direction, heading right for where I should be heading. But all of a sudden I began to veer, not mildly, but wildly to the left. Since I thought that the bus would be waiting for me directly across the street, I listened for its sound. The motor of a bus is very distinctive, and it is a good guide. I felt it should be to the right of me as I crossed, but it appeared to be to the left of me, so I thought I was making a poor crossing and veered to the left. All of a sudden I was startled by a car passing in front of me. No car was supposed to be there! Then I was even more shocked by a car whizzing behind me.

In a flash I realized what was wrong. My bus was standing on the side street, and I had not needed to make any correction at all. Now I would have to make a correction in the opposite direction to get back there. But here I was in the midst of traffic, and it was perilous to move in any direction at all. Fortunately there was a Good Samaritan on the street corner. He was a Good Samaritan right out of the Scriptures; he was deaf, and had an impediment in his speech. When I tried to tell him what I wanted to do, he could not understand me. When he told me what he was going to do, I could not understand him. But he swept me boldly and safely through all that traffic to the corner opposite from where my bus was waiting. I was safe, but as I stood there, I heard the bus roar and pull off. I had missed it. Bob came over laughing and asking me what in the world I had done. When I explained to him, he could see what I had been thinking about and said that wasn't so bad, but he also warned, "Be sure that you get the exact directions from the bus company as to what corner the bus is on. Get the name of the street and the geographic location, northeast, southeast, or whatever it may be." And so I had learned a lesson.

Meanwhile at the Center, my work with Braille proceeded slowly. My education did give me an advantage in that I could guess at words even if I sometimes could not read them. Some of the students could read a word—they could find the letters that made up the word with their fingers—but then they could not recognize it as a word because of their poor education. My problem was that my fingers were not very sensitive. At last, though, the time came when I was able to do many of the things with Braille that I had always wanted to do. I can now read the devotional booklet, *Portals of Prayer,* with considerable ease. I can read the Bible with some readiness, and I can make notes for meetings that I can read in the meeting. I can also read Braille while lying flat on my back simply putting the book on my chest. I didn't think the time would ever come when I would be able to do this. Some very fine Christian people at St. John's offered to buy me a Braille Bible, which cost one hundred dollars, and I gratefully accepted their offer. The Bible consists of eighteen volumes, fourteen for the Old Testament and four for the New Testament, and it takes up about four feet on my book shelf. The handicap of a Braille Bible is that if you want to carry it back and forth to church, you have to know which volumes you want to use. Actually, I use it mostly for study at home and seldom take it to church. I still memorize the passages that I want to use in the Sunday morning service. And with the King James Version on records, the Today's English Version on tape, and the Revised Standard Version in Braille, I feel that I am somewhat equipped again for studying the Scriptures and doing my work.

Every time I returned to the Center from my ten days at Midland, I was oppressed by the feeling that the young people there, as well as some of the older ones, were so far short of finding a place for themselves in life. I had something that I could always turn to. The Center was merely an episode in my life. I was definitely preparing myself for better and greater service in my ministry. But these people would have difficult times finding a place in society. Some students had hopes of becoming medical transcriptionists because they were very good at typing. Others planned to go to Cleveland and take courses that would fit them for taking care of vending machines in government buildings. Others intended to go on to college. Some might become social workers and others wanted to work with occupational therapy. But many of the young people had neither the ability nor the inner urge to improve their situation. They would simply drift into living on a pension for the blind and would make little of their lives. The Center exerted itself to rouse these people, but required cooperation from parents at home and from other agencies also. For some blind people it is simply a difficult thing to get away from family and home and to face an entirely new world with all sorts of challenges.

I continued to try to arrange ways in which the young people at the Center could get in touch with sighted young people and exchange viewpoints with them. It was not only that I wanted the blind people to get a better look at the outside world, but I wanted the young people from the University to appreciate the situation of the blind. Since, as we have said, a number of young people from St. John's were going to Western, I invited them one by one, or two by two, and we set up a number of dinner parties.

The Center itself also provided various activities for its students. They arranged bowling parties, swimming parties, and various other expeditions. Bowling could be accomplished with the assistance of a rack supplied by the bowling alley, a metal track which the blind person could take hold of as he strode down the alley and which would guide him toward the proper place for releasing the ball. Swimming, too, was enjoyable, but it had its hazards. When we went to the YWCA pool, we found that there was a rope down the center of the pool, and we could swim down each side of that, but we had to keep on going in the proper direction so we would not run into traffic coming from the other way. The pool was reserved just for the blind during that time so we had no particular problems, but I found out it was difficult to keep contact with the rope. I could become confused without too much difficulty and get all the way turned around if I once lost contact. It was enjoyable, though, to get this exercise and stretch my legs a little. There was the usual horseplay—the boys trying to find the girls and shoving them, tickling them, or upsetting them.

During evenings at the Center, the most common recreation was listening to records in the cafeteria. Quite a number of the young people had albums of their favorite music, and sometimes there was quite a rush after supper to see who would be the first to play a particular album on the record player. Generally the younger people took care of the record player until far into the evening, but sometimes I would come down later and put on some of my records. Occasionally, a few of the young people would stop in and listen, even though it was late at night. Then someone would say, "Wouldn't it be nice if we had a pizza?" And that was the signal for calling up the pizza place. We would feast on pizza and perhaps a can of pop from the vending machine as late as 11:30 and everybody was in a gay mood.

Meal time was often an occasion for various types of hilarity. The meals were generally good, and there were occasions when everybody looked forward to a special treat. Cream puff day was one of these, and on one particular cream puff day, one of the boys, Andy, who had a way with the cooks, managed to procure for himself two cream puffs. All during the meal he gloated over the fact that he had two cream puffs and was going to have a feast. However, his gloating goaded some of the girls and fellows at his table to the point where they felt that he should suffer a little. They quietly spirited away his cream puffs and hid them at the end of the table. When Andy's great moment came, all he could do was let out a baleful lament, "Who stole my cream puffs?"

Everybody at the table pleaded innocence, but Andy

persisted. Meanwhile, one of the girls had eaten the filling from her cream puff, but left the shell, so this shell was given to Andy and he was asked if he were blind or something. He reached out, found the cream puff, and said, "Now I am going to eat." A moment later he bellowed again, "Who stole the stuffing out of my cream puff?"

They slipped one of the cream puffs back in front of his plate and said, "What's the matter with you, Andy? You've got a cream puff there."

He reached out and found the cream puff. Then he let go of it to feel for the other one, and somebody slid the first cream puff away. Again Andy screamed, "Who stole my cream puffs?"

Then someone asked him, "Andy, have you had your hearing test here at the Center yet? Can't you tell when one of your cream puffs is disappearing?"

He hollered, "There's nothing wrong with my hearing. Who can hear good enough to tell when a cream puff is taking off?"

Finally his tormentors relented; Andy got his cream puffs, and peace reigned again in the dining room.

One of the ways of finding a little recreation at the Center was to take a walk along the bicycle track if the weather was not too inclement, and I used to ask various people to take a turn with me. One afternoon a girl by the name of Sherry and I went out. But after thirty or forty feet we got into a little altercation about who was to be the guide on this particular trip. We each had our cane, and it is difficult for both to use their canes going around the circle if they really want to walk together. One person has to shoulder his cane and take the arm of the other. We got into a sort of tug of war over each other's canes, and we pulled each other this way and that until we pulled each other off of the bicycle track onto the grass and finally into the ditch alongside the track. We got up laughing, and I can't even remember who was the winner. But there was a Scriptural moral to this: "Can the blind lead the blind? shall they not both fall into the ditch?" (Luke 6:39)

Much of what went on at the Center at this time was a "marking of time," a slow gathering of experience in working with the blind, understanding the blind, and so understanding other handicapped people. For me it was a living with other people until I had gained certain talents and experiences that would be helpful in my work at St. John's

One thing that I had taken up was gym. Because of my age, I was not requred to do so, but I wanted to because I did not get much exercise, and I rather enjoyed various activities, the bicycle, rowing maching, weight lifting, etc. Another elective I took was the course in abacus. The abacus had always intrigued me, particularly because I had no idea how the thing worked. I found out that it was relatively simple, that the mental calculations were not the difficult part, for me it was again my big, awkward fingers pushing the beads into their proper positions. After I had become more adept at handling the beads, I found out that I could manage most of the computations without much trouble.

There was also a course in Home Repairs, in which we had to repair faucets, switches, and sockets on lamps. We also had to clean out the drain of the bathtub and learn to paint with a roller over a certain area. Many of the things that have to be done around the house were covered in this course, and it was quite valuable. The purpose of all this, of course, was to drive home the point that a blind person can do most anything if he sets his mind to it and perhaps has a little special equipment to help him and once in a while a word of advice from some person who is sighted.

In the Techniques of Daily Living Class, we worked at making beds, dusting, cleaning the bathroom, wiping up windows, and various kinds of cooking: frying an egg, scrambling an egg, frying bacon in a press, making a cake, making tea and coffee, and pouring hot drinks. There are various ways to pour coffee—for example, simply by listening to the sound of the coffee as it comes into the cup. The best way, we were told, was to put your finger over the edge of the cup until you felt the hot coffee. This was something that you did in the kitchen, though. You did not use this particular system before the eyes of the drinkers. Some of the students particularly liked cooking. Even some of the older men took to making casseroles and things of this kind and they brought them to the cafeteria where they distributed them among their friends. Everyone wanted to hear words of praise about his particular concoction and, of course, all of these things were a welcome addition to the usual menu. On these occasions the diabetics often sneaked a cookie or a piece of cake from somebody's offering without the cooks knowing about it.

In the room devoted to Aural and Oral Arts, we not only learned how to operate various types of tape recorders and other equipment, but we learned how to dub in on tapes, to use patch cords, to use two tape recorders at one time, and to put several things on a tape in sequence. We were even encouraged to experiment. Some people produced little radio shows, others had little plays or dramas. My contribution was a religious article on the Lord's Prayer in which I managed to squeeze some English, German, Latin, and Greek just to show off my Liberal Arts education and training for the ministry. We became acquainted with a specially modified version of the Sony tape recorder and player that had been designed for use by blind people and also had some experiments with compressed speech, what it was and what uses it might be put. Generally, compressed speech was difficult for us, and we did not enjoy listening to it. It required intense concentration and did not seem in the end to be worth it.

Occupational Therapy was never my favorite subject. I did not enjoy sewing on a button or sewing together a seam or putting on, after several false attempts, a snap. I also had difficulty with the Technique of Eating Program where we had to work with plastic or modeling-clay steak and plastic corn, peas, and beans, to practice eating them in the proper way. All this was a little bit boring.

But I would not only "mark time," amuse myself, and gain new experiences in personal relationships. Some real pastoral, ministerial work was in store for me among these people.

Chapter 7
Targets of Opportunity

The work that really intrigued me at the Center, outside of the courses I had come particularly to master, Mobility and Braille, was the opportunity for counseling that came up under so many conditions and on so many occasions. Although I generally had little to do with the weekly Bible class—I did not like to interfere with the man who was in charge of it, had been for a long time, and would be after I was gone—there was one occasion when he was not able to be present and I did take over the class. Circumstances led to an unusual discussion. I had selected a passage that I knew pretty well by heart, because my Braille was not good enough for me to read it out of the Bible and a Christian woman who had written a book on the blind was to be with us. Just before I went to the class, I had a long distance telephone call from Clara. She told me that one of our students from St. John's, who had been attending Michigan State University—a young man whom I knew very well and with whose family I was closely associated—had been stabbed to death by two assailants while crossing the campus late in the evening. There seemed to be no motive for the crime. The young man had been able to get to the roadway and find help. He was taken to the hospital where he was able to give some account, but he soon died because of the number and depth of the stab wounds.

This was a shocking thing to me, and I brought it with me into the class that night. I had pretty well forgotten the text which I had prepared, and we discussed the fact that things like this can happen in the world in which we live.

We know that God watches over us, and God was watching over this young man, and yet something like this could happen. We talked a great deal about why these things happen; that we live in a sinful world; that this is a place where the prince of this world, the devil, has much power, but that when these things happen the gracious and forgiving God is still standing by; and even if we lose our lives, eternal salvation is forever ours. The atmosphere that arose in the class after I told them what I had heard on the telephone was a very somber one, and we discussed various things, pointing out particularly the vulnerability of blind people. Blind people are advised always to have some money with them, as much as $10, so if at any time they are attacked, if any time they are robbed—like perhaps by a drug-crazed person—they will not be submitted to injury or death simply because the drug-crazed person is disappointed not to find any money. The $10 will generally satisfy a person in that state, and it is a cheap price to pay for not being assaulted or not being murdered.

The story of this murder made a deep impression upon us because we realized that if things like this could happen to sighted people, they could happen much more easily to people who are not sighted. The Center itself was an island of safety—we felt no concerns there—but the world outside is for many blind people a very dangerous place.

Opportunities for counseling came from many unexpected directions. One day a young black asked me if he could talk to me privately. I said certainly, and so we went into the library which was often unoccupied. This young man was all worked up because he felt he was not being treated fairly by his counselor. But as I listened to his story, I realized that there were certainly two sides to it. The young man had his feelings about certain matters, and it was evident that the counselor had found it necessary to speak to him rather plainly about his attitude, and he resented this.

Of course, it is not the business of a counselor to simply

be friends with the person whom he is counseling. It is his duty to point out places where the person is going astray, mistakes he is making, and things which are holding him back from his own development. One can become very unpopular even when he presents these things in the most tactful way. This young black man was resenting what his counselor was telling him, and after I had listened to him for a while I told him that he should realize that his counselor had no reason for not treating him fairly. I said that this was one of the temptations to which black people were put and that they shouldn't feel that white people are necessarily against them. It was to the advantage of the white counselor to do the best job that he possibly could with the person whom he was counseling. I pointed out that some of the things which the counselor had said could be good advice.

"If you are really a wise and clever fellow," I said, "you have to look at how much truth there is in some of the things that he has said to you. He's only pointing these things out, not to make fun of you but because he wants you to be as good, as happy, and as successful a person in this world as you can be. If some of the things you are doing are keeping you from becoming that, you ought to listen to him."

The young man finally agreed that he would not lose his temper, nor would he make a complaint to the director of the institution. Instead he was going to go along with the counselor and listen to what he had to say. I don't know just exactly what the final relationship was between the counselor and the counselee, but I do know that a good relationship developed between this young man and me. Some time later he invited me to go out to dinner with him and his girl friend, and a year or so after I had left the Center, I received a message from him through a young man of our congregation who had happened to meet him in the town where he was working.

At this time the original thorn in the flesh began to give me a few scratches. My right eye began to water and cause pain. I went to the doctor who served the Institution in Kalamzaoo, Dr. Skutt, and he examined the eye, could not determine what was wrong with it, and told me to come back in about a week. However, that next week I was back in Midland and when I decided to consult my doctor there, I found that he was not in. When later I decided to return to Kalamazoo, the eye was not troubling me so much and I let it ride, although generally in the mornings it caused me considerable pain and difficulty. But at the other times of the day it gave me very little problem. So it was something I found that I could live with, if I could just get through the hours of the morning when it was most uncomfortable.

When I finally got back to see my doctor in Midland, it was very close to the time when I was ready to stay there permanently again, and he diagnosed the problem as glaucoma. This is a complication that often follows a diabetic retinopathy, and it has the disadvantage of being very painful because it is a pressure that builds up in the eye. The doctor began a series of treatments through various types of drops, but eventually I paid the price, probably for my neglect, with an operation.

One day another young man approached me and said he would like to talk to me privately. We found a corner and he told me that he and his girl friend, who was also a student at the Center, had gone out that previous weekend and stayed with a relative. This gave them an opportunity for a passionate relationship in which he said they went very far, so far, in fact, that his girl friend might have become pregnant. What bothered him was that he now felt that he had a different feeling toward the girl. He didn't know whether he loved her any more or not.

Well, I chided him a bit at first by telling him that he knew he had gone too far, and that what he was feeling now was part of the penalty which a person had to pay for an excess of this kind. When our relationship depends too much upon the sexual instead of the other things which bind us together, it will fade and its strength becomes less obvious, and we become confused about how we really feel toward one another. Much would depend on how this girl felt toward him, and they would simply have to continue their relationship for a while to see if they could rebuild it on a proper basis. It would be a matter of asking God's direction and God's help, asking forgiveness for a sin, and at the same time looking at each other in real love, desiring the real welfare of the other person and not just the satisfaction of one's personal desires.

I had great sympathy for this young couple, because I think that perhaps blind young people are prone to become quite passionate in their relationships. After all, when the blind young man and young woman meet each other, they cannot gauge each other by sight. The blind person depends upon what he hears and also his sense of touch, so that caresses become very important to him, not simply as a gesture of love, but also as a way of learning what the other person actually looks like. There's a temptation in these relationships to do what is described somewhat vulgarly as "Brailling a girl out," and sometimes young people holler this at each other when they meet a new acquaintance. They shake hands with a girl, and someone says, "Okay, Braille her out!" It's proper to place one's hands upon the face of the other person, also upon the shoulders and perhaps the waist. Thus one can have some conception of what the person is like. But two young blind people who want to become better acquainted with each other are very likely to become better acquainted by embracing, by exploring each other physically, and this can lead to temptation.

The Center apparently sometimes had to accept students who had psychiatric problems, and it was not always clear at the outset whether they could really be of much help to these students or not. It depended upon the depth of their problem. On one occasion a student came who was so quiet that conversation with him was hardly possible. He had no contact with the other students. Very little could be accomplished in class, except perhaps in the Occupational Therapy Department. At the same time he had very unusual talents. He could sit beside the television set when the baseball game was in progress and describe the action that was taking place there, the play-by-play account, in a way that would have done credit to any sports broadcaster. One could hardly realize that he was blind and had probably never seen a game. There was no contact on my part with this particular student except that twice I accidentally picked up his cane from the cafeteria and caused him to dissolve in a rage of frustrated tears. The Center could do little for this person, and so he was only with us for several weeks.

Sometimes members of the staff at the Center would come to me and ask about things. One of the men on the staff had had a particularly unhappy divorce and was desolate about it. One day he poured out the whole story of his unhappiness and all the terrible things he had gone through. It was dreadful to hear a man so distressed, and I could not know, of course, to what extent he had been at fault in the marriage and to what extent his wife had been at fault. However, I could counsel him that this extremity was a time to turn to God for the consolation that He always has for us. If he was at fault in any way in this marriage, forgiveness was available to him through Jesus Christ, and in the bleak outlook that lay before him, he should realize that God could still bring joy and peace into his life. This seemed to impress him, and he said that he was by all means going to go to church and get the spiritual encouragement which he now realized that he needed.

One night, one of the nurses on duty began to talk to me about various religious questions. She belonged to a church and was interested in religion, so we started to talk at about 11 o'clock. Alberta happened to be sitting with us, and from time to time she chimed in. When the nurse had to make a round, I waited up for her because our discussion was not over. Alberta decided that she did not want to go to bed either. She said that she had never stayed up all night in her life, and for once she wanted to do it. Well, it was a Friday night, and the nurse and I humored her. Not until 5 o'clock did we realize we had talked the subject out. This was only a part of the religious discussions which we were to have with this nurse, and it led to a very pleasant relationship between us.

I also had frequent discussions with Jan, the girl who had led our jingle bell expedition. She was in her later twenties, and had a great deal of difficulty in deciding what she wanted to do. She was partly sighted, yet she was very good in Braille. In fact, she did Braille transcriptions, but this is not very profitable work. The pay is meager, and the time consumed and amount of concentration required in order to keep these transcriptions error-free is great. So Jan did them only with reluctance. She had trouble sometimes with her parents wanting her to do one thing and other relatives feeling that she should do another thing, but her religious beliefs helped keep her cheerful. I was sorry that I could never help resolve the problem of what she wanted to do with her life. Possibly it was an insoluble one at the time because she did not get exactly the support that she needed from her parents, nor could she in her own mind decide just how far it was possible for her to go in college or in training for any special work.

Again and again, as I talked with Jan, I was grateful that I had work to do, and it brought home to me again the plight of the blind person who has so little opportunity and must work very hard to make use of such opportunity as comes to him. Often employers are reluctant to hire a blind person. They think immediately of responsibility. What if the blind person is injured? What if he makes mistakes? The blind person properly trained for a particular job is as capable generally as a sighted person, except in certain situations. But the blind person also knows what situations he cannot enter into and even in a matter like woodworking, using a power saw or an electric sander, he knows precisely what he can do and cannot do, and is as safe in his work as a sighted person would be. In fact, he knows that he cannot afford to make a mistake and is more conscious of this than the sighted person, who sometimes cuts off a finger simply because he is careless. There is much work to be done in persuading employers, unions, and all sorts of people that the blind person can be a trusted and valued employee in many types of work.

Alberta also had problems which she liked to discuss from time to time. Sometimes it was boyfriends. There were young men, blind men, who came and called on her, wanted to take her out, who telephoned her, and who apparently had serious intentions toward her, but she was not entranced with any of them. She had either set her sights higher or they just were not simply the type of person that she could think of marrying. Instead, she looked forward to the summer camp to which she was going the following summer.

"In that camp," she said, "I'll meet lots of young people, and that's where I'm going to pick up my boyfriend."

Alberta also had difficulty trying to decide what she wanted to do. She was sent downtown to take various kinds of tests and despised most of them. Either because of her attitude toward them or because of her lack of facility with them, nothing much came of the tests. I think the tests showed certain things she could do, but she was not particularly anxious to do them. Finally she had to leave the Center, for they had done everything they could for her. It was up to her counselor in Grand Rapids to help her along the next step.

I also had a plan which I thought might work out in the case of a presentable girl like Alberta. A young blind person could come into a Christian church, such as St. John's, stay there for a week and work with the children in the parish school, the nursery school children, the Sunday school children, the Bible class children, the Sunday services, the devotions on Wednesday, and the various meetings that went on during the week. The blind person could be paid for this and a double benefit would accrue. The blind person would have an opportunity to show capabilities and earn money, and the congregation would be opened up to the realization that blind people are people with whom one can get along, carry on conversations, and have a good time. More about this later.

I learned some things from Alberta too. I learned, for example, that people who have been blind since birth and who have started learning Braille when they were perhaps five years old, may have a very good knowledge of Braille but none of the English alphabet. They have no idea what the letter "A" is like or the letter "B," either in small letters or in capitals. This came to light when a middle-aged man, who was blind, deaf, and dumb, appeared at the Center. He knew Braille, but his means of communication was through palm writing. This meant that you would hold out your palm, and he would inscribe letters upon it—English letters, generally capitals. If he went slowly he could write on my palm, and I could understand what he was writing. Alberta became interested in this man, and he in her. But she could make nothing of the writing that he did on her palm, and since she was so confused, I explained that he was writing regular letters, the letters of the English language, capital letters. She said, "Well, I don't know what they are."

I then found out that practically none of the students, even the very brightest, knew what the English alphabet looks like. So I went ahead and tried to teach them. I tried to tell them that an "A" was composed of a five and nine leaning against each other—with a little "c" connecting the two in the middle. They were acquainted with these things, and this sometimes was a way of getting them to visualize something that they could not visualize otherwise. We did make progress with this, and eventually Alberta learned enough letters of the alphabet so that she could communicate with the man.

Certain other students also became interested in palm writing and asked me to help them to learn the letters of the alphabet. For eighteen years of their lives they had had no occasion to use the letters of the alphabet, but now there seemed to be some purpose; at least they could communicate with a deaf and dumb person.

Some time in February a young woman called Helen arrived at the Center and became a challenge to my every pastoral instinct. She was a very beautiful girl, but had problems. She showed what amounted to almost genius in getting off on the wrong foot with the student body when at the first meal, she proclaimed that she very much liked boys, liked to kiss them, and furthermore was going to "save" every person at the Center.

I had my first contact with Helen one day in the OT room. My instructor had insisted that I must do some sort of leather work, and so I finally chose to work on a scabbard for my slate and stylus. This involved tying with a thin strand of leather, and it was hard sledding for an old fumble-fingers like myself. I had to do some of the work over and over again, but after some three weeks of working on it five days a week, I managed to finish my master work and bring it to my teacher for her approval. Lest I become overly proud with my magnificent accomplishment, she said to me, "Well, it's okay. But it took you fifteen hours. Helen here can do it in one hour." Since at that time I shared the common conviction that Helen was a girl of little talent, this was very close to being an insult. But I did get acquainted with Helen.

One thing she frequently did was to go into the game room, sit down, and play the piano. This caused some disharmony with the rest of the student body because there were some others that liked to play the piano also, and the competition for time at the instrument was sometimes quite strong. There was also a great difference between the kind of music which Helen played and the others played. Some of the others played popular music, and some improvised, but Helen played a strictly religious music, some Gospel-type, and also ordinary hymns. I was surprised that she could play many, many melodies without any music, just from having heard them in church. I rather admired her ability but found that in only a few cases did she know the words that went with the music. So I would sometimes sit down and sing the words as she played. One day she said, "Would you teach me some of the words to this music?"

I said, "Sure." And I began to teach her by rote. One day we even went into the Braille room. She was quite adept at typing on the Braille writer, and I dictated a number of songs such as "I know that my Redeemer lives," "Just as I am, without one plea," and "My faith looks up to Thee," which she could memorize at her leisure. This gave her a great deal of pleasure and caused her to form a bond of attachment to me. I wasn't aware of it immediately, but I soon became a sort of father image to her, and she began to seek me out.

One day I happened to have my tape recorder with me, and as she played and sang I made a recording. When she had finished I asked her if she would like to hear what she sounded like.

She said, "Oh, did you make a tape of my playing?"

I said, "Yes." So I played it back to her and she was intrigued. Again and again she would ask me if I would tape another piece for her.

One day she said, "I wish you'd bring your tape recorder and we'll just sit down and talk into it." I found out this was for her a type of play-acting that was quite revealing. When she spoke to the tape recorder she spoke about herself and not as she was but as she would like to be apparently—a married woman with a child who had some problems. I was to play the part of a Roman Catholic priest with whom she could discuss these problems. I was amused at this but went along and what was revealed gave me great compassion for the inner conflicts that went on within her mind, the things which she felt she could not attain, and would like to attain, and the hopes, sometimes unreasonable, that she desired to fulfill.

In certain relationships she was very naive. Sometimes she would speak about boys. She said she liked to have them kiss her, but they always wanted to do other things which she didn't like.

I said, "Well, if they do things that you don't like, what do you say to them?"

She said, "I tell them I would rather not have them do that to me."

I laughed and said, "You have to go farther than that. This is one time when you can use some strong language if you want to. This is the time when you can be violent and slap somebody, because you have to be very firm with people. Boys will be boys, and you have to protect yourself."

I was never quite sure whether some of the experiences which she related were fact or fantasy. Sometimes her father image of me tended to swerve into that of a boyfriend, and she would ask me, "How old are you? Can you be my boyfriend?"

And I would say, "No. We can just be Christian friends. People who believe in Christ and who like to talk together and do things together can be Christian friends without being anything more than that."

She seemed to accept that, and this was one of the reasons why later on she went to church with me at Zion. She behaved herself very well, and I introduced her to the pastors there in the hope that they could be of help to her after I had left the Center, which I soon planned to do.

The general attitude which the other students had toward Helen caused me to think of her as an underdog, and I went out of my way to befriend her. She had gotten in the habit of sitting by herself at a table in the dining hall, so I would make it a point to go over and sit with her, sometimes deserting the friends which I would have preferred to have been sitting with. She was very happy about this, and we got along well.

Since she had great difficulty in giving her attention to anything for an extended period of time, she could hardly compose letters, and it was even hard for her to speak to her mother on the telephone. I used to encourage her to do this. Sometimes she refused to even answer the telephone if her mother was on the line. On one occasion she was to make some sort of a presentation in a class, and I had to get her to type one sentence on a piece of paper, then force her to think on to the next statement, get that on paper, and so on till she had something acceptable.

Gradually Helen was accepted more and more by the other young people, and took part in a group of three or four that did some play-acting almost every evening. There was a fellow by the name of Jim who liked to do imitations and was rather good at it. He needed stooges for this, and had a number of girls who enjoyed taking part, one of whom was Helen. She was very proud of the fact that she was included in this group, and every evening they sat down at one of the tables and carried on.

However, one day when I was in the cafeteria, I heard the other members of the group discussing Helen and deriding her very strongly in such a way that I almost protested because they were not only being unkind, they were being slanderous as young people sometimes will be. The next evening some sort of altercation arose at their evening play-acting, and when I happened to come into the lounge, Jim was demanding that Helen give him an apology. Helen was crying and complaining that she didn't see any reason why she should apologize.

I went up to Jim and said, "Listen, you just about spoiled my meal the other day by talking about Helen the way you did—you and the other girls here—and I think if any apologies should be given, you ought to apologize to her for the way you talked about her."

He was much taken aback at this, and since I had raised my voice I had the attention of the whole group. The quiet was broken by Helen's wailing and the tears of the other girls who were involved and who began to have feelings of bad conscience. This sort of cleared the air, though. There were apologies and things went on as before.

Once in a while Helen would express particularly appealing ideas. As we took a little walk around the track one day, she asked if I thought that God knew that every time she went outside she talked with the birds and that the birds talked back to her in their own language. I said I was sure that since God knew everything He knew this also.

After I left the Center, I telephoned a number of times to see how Helen was getting along. About the second or third time she said, "Oh, I have a boyfriend now, and everything is going along well." I'm sure that this was not a solution to her problems, but it was probably the best that she could expect for some time to come.

As Easter approached even these many opportunities I had for counseling—and I have mentioned only a few of them—faded into insignificance as I contemplated my desire to be back with St. John's and take part in the services in Holy Week. I, therefore, had to concentrate on all the things which I was doing. I had to get up a little earlier and stay up a little later to finish my Braille assignments and prepare for a comprehensive examination that I would take before I left. In Mobility, Bob Hall stepped up the pace and handed me a number of rather difficult assignments.

Spring was in the air and the weather was warming up. I knew that the crocuses would be blooming on the south side of our house, and I was anxious to get back. I could no longer see them, but their coming always intrigued me every spring. Before I knew it, the last week at the Center was at hand, and after Bob Hall had done his worst with me, I sat down on the last day for a three-hour test that covered everything I had taken in Braille. My eye was troubling me again and I had difficulty concentrating. Since Braille requires great concentration, a three-hour test is asking a little too much, but I was able to give sufficient evidence that I had studied well and absorbed a great deal of what I was expected to know.

On that very day Clara descended and in a few minutes we gathered up my baggage and, hardly saying good-bye to anybody, took off for Midland. Most of the people with whom I had been intimately acquainted had already left the Center. New people were coming in, and suddenly I felt like a stranger among strange people.

It seemed like there should have been some feeling of transition between leaving the Center and coming back to St. John's, but there wasn't, partly because I had been coming back so often and partly because it was the beginning of Holy Week. There would be services on Wednesday, Thursday, Friday afternoon, and Friday evening. There would be services on Easter Sunday at sunrise, an Easter breakfast, and then two other services later in the morning. Activity would be at a peak. And right after Easter, we would concentrate on the confirmation class, a group of probably fifty young people, ages thirteen to fourteen, that would be confirmed on the first Sunday in May. I also felt an overwhelming desire to catch up on all the prospects, all the contacts which had been made during the preceding months. This was my specialty, and I wanted to be on with it.

Nevertheless, in spite of all these things, I wanted to carry out a plan which I had been developing for some time—that of having a blind person come into the congregation for a week. I had already made contact with Alberta, and she agreed to spend about ten days in Midland. We would pay her for this, and she would have no expenses whatever. We would even see to it that she had transportation to and from Grand Rapids. This was arranged for the latter part of April, and I wrote to the District Board of Social Ministry, telling them about my plans, which they encouraged me to carry out. They even offered to send—and did send—two young women from Concordia Junior College in Ann Arbor who were preparing themselves for work in sociology. They would observe what we were trying to do. Clara and I also planned our annual drivers' and readers' banquet for the week that Alberta would be here.

Toward the end of April, Clara and I made the trip to Grand Rapids, picked up Alberta, and spirited her off to Midland. She would stay at our house.

Alberta had a pleasing way of visiting the various classrooms in our parish school. She would explain to the lower grades that at night she went to her room, got ready for bed, lay down on the bed, and then she took her book, put it on her stomach, and read herself to sleep. The children were intrigued with the fact that a blind person could read in the dark, could read herself to sleep without having to hold a book up, by simply letting it rest on her stomach and feeling the letters. Alberta had brought along books with pictures outlined by Braille dots. The children were mystified by these, especially when they were told that the dots were letters and words. Alberta would then, either with her slate and stylus or with the Braille writer, write down their names on pieces of paper. She also showed them what the Braille letters were and how to use a Braille writer. We had some cards on which the Braille alphabet was written, and the children cherished these and had a lot of pleasure out of them. But mainly they became accustomed to a blind person. They were not shy or diffident. They knew that you could speak to a blind person just like you spoke to anyone else.

Alberta did similar things in the Sunday school, the nursery school, the kindergarten, and in gatherings such as the young people's group. When Sunday morning came, we made her the center of attraction. She appeared at the church services and read both the Gospel and the Epistle, flawlessly, amazing everybody who didn't realize that a blind person who has been trained from youth can read Braille as fluently as the sighted person can read print. At the end of each of the services Alberta and I also put on a display for the congregation, showing the technique of using the cane, how to sight-guide a person, and how to give directions. We also pointed out some of the do's and don'ts of how to help people who are blind—and when not to help them. I particularly spoke about my chief peeve that people always try to open the door of a car for me. We had a door offering after each service to pay the honorarium that we had promised Alberta, and were really overwhelmed when it amounted to much more than we needed or expected.

During the week that followed, we again had Alberta go to each of the classrooms in the parish school. This meant that she was busy every morning, but afternoons were hers and the evenings were generally filled with some sort of a meeting or group that she was to attend. One evening she went to the home of one of our members who had open house for young people, and they had an opportunity to meet with her, although we found that it was a little difficult for them to speak freely with her. But possibly this was because young people tend to gather in their little groups and cliques, and any stranger would have had some difficulty in breaking into these circles, whether blind or not.

Some afternoons Alberta and I went out on walks to practice our cane technique. She had little opportunity to practice in the little suburb of Belmont where she lived because there were very few sidewalks, and it really takes a concrete sidewalk or something of that nature to use your cane technique to best advantage.

Once we ran into something that the person who uses a cane always has to be aware of, a low-hanging branch. There are usually city ordinances which make it necessary for property owners to trim their trees in such a way that the branches do not hang too low over sidewalks, but sometimes in the spring the growth of the trees causes new branches to hang down before the owners can get around to trimming them. I had the misfortune to run smack into one of these limbs, a limb that was over an inch thick. Alberta had safely passed underneath it because she was shorter than I, but it caught me right across the eye. I was so incensed that I grabbed the branch and tried to break it off, but it was too limber.

The property owner came out and, looking at my eye said, "You'd better go see a doctor. Your eye is bleeding." I put my fingers up to my eye and felt the wetness there. We were only about two blocks from home, and when we reached there we found Clara home ahead of us, which was fortunate. Well, not exactly, for when Clara saw the eye she almost swooned. At least she screeched and did a few other things because of the blood that was running from the eyelid. So I took a trip to the emergency entrance of the hospital where six stitches were taken in my eyelid, and no further damage resulted except some temporary discomfort.

Alberta and I also relived some days at the Center by sitting up and listening to records and eating this, that, and the other as suited our fancy. When Wednesday came, she took part in the parish school devotions and also put on a demonstration of the cane technique for them, which was well received. Thursday was the day for the readers' and drivers' banquet, and again Alberta was the star performer.

This Thursday evening party was the climax of Alberta's stay, and the next day we whisked her off again to Grand Rapids. The two young girls who had been present while Alberta was with us sent in a fine report to the Board of Social Ministry. The Board was much interested in the project, but when I tried to approach Alberta about doing this sort of thing on a regular basis, or doing it once or twice a month, she felt that she could not. It was one thing for her to come to St. Johns' where she knew me and my wife but an entirely different thing to come to a church where she knew nobody, in surroundings which were altogether foreign to her. Though I urged her, she still refused. I toyed with the idea of perhaps finding other suitable girls, but the Board of Social Ministry said that since the difficulty was to find the right girl, they did not see how the program could be brought forward any further. So the matter was dropped.

About a year later, Pastor Lionel Skanser of Faith church in Bay City invited me to come over, preach about the blind and handicapped, and give a program similar to that which I had given at St. John's. There was a blind girl in his congregation with whom I could work as I had with

Alberta. She read the Gospel and the Epistle, I preached, and we gave a demonstration of cane technique after the service. I also spoke to the Bible class about the Center and about the problems of the blind people. We had a very pleasant morning, and apparently the congregation enjoyed this too.

Although the idea that I had developed to have someone like Alberta go from church to church on a regular schedule did not mature, I found other ways in which I could further the cause of the blind. At the Spring Conference that year I asked for a few moments of the Conference's time and spoke to this group briefly about blind people and the difficulties under which many of them labored. I encouraged every pastor to check out his congregation to see how many blind people he had and to be sure they were getting the best use of the things which the State made available. The address was well received and bore fruit almost immediately. I began to receive invitations to speak at Lutheran Laymen's League rallies, Lutheran Women's Missionary League gatherings, meetings of men's clubs and women's societies. Perhaps it was these things that first showed me that the blindness with which I had been stricken was not a hindrance to my ministry but a furtherance of it. I had not only been able to continue to work in my own church, but I had rallied the people around me in a fellowship and association which was something good and beneficial for them, for me, and for the church at large. Now simply because I was a blind person, I was enabled to go out and speak to groups everywhere, always having a Christian message but also able to put forth the cause of the blind.

The type of addresses which I developed for these occasions were generally quite light in the sense that I made jokes and introduced some of the ridiculous things that can happen to a blind person. So there was a great deal of laughter in connection with my presentations as well as some very earnest and sincere thoughts about the situation of the blind, the importance of religion in their lives, and the importance of their having assistance from Christian people everywhere.

On one occasion I attended a meeting of the Lions' Club which sponsors a leader dog training program and is very proud of this. I happened to speak in this program about the fact that I have a fine group of drivers, mostly women, who serve me so wonderfully in this capacity. I laid it on very thick, saying that our requirements were very strict for this group. "They have to be beautiful, intelligent, good conversationalists, and they have to drive Cadillacs." After I had told them all about the wonders of this fine group of people that supported me, somebody got up and asked the question, "Have you ever thought about having a leader dog?"

I stopped as if I had been shocked, and said, "Sir, after I have told you all about this wonderful group of beautiful ladies, you want me to trade them all for a dog?"

Then, of course, I went on to explain that a dog would not be very helpful to me in my present situation, since I must sometimes drive miles between calls. I must make many calls in hospitals and nursing homes, and it is difficult sometimes to handle a dog under such circumstances, especially when you stay there for several hours as I often do. Also, there is the problem of taking care of a dog which I noticed was a difficult one for some of the people at the Center. The dog must be fed, cleaned, and exercised, and a strict discipline must be maintained, which is sometimes rather difficult.

One day I wrote to Rev. Walter Storm, executive secretary of The Lutheran Church—Missouri Synod's board for work among the blind, and asked him if there was anything that I could do in my position as a blind pastor to further the work of the blind in our Synod. At this time the Synod was contenting itself with providing Braille materials. The core, the devotional booklet *Portals of Prayer*, was reproduced in Braille free of charge for any blind person. That means that a little book, which is about four by six, comes out in a Braille edition which is about fifteen by twelve and as thick as a small telephone book. Synod's board for the blind also prints magazines of a religious nature, such as *The Lutheran Messenger*, and other religious materials, and maintains an office in St. Louis, Missouri. On the whole, work among the blind in the church is different from work among the deaf. The deaf, for example, have to have a special type of ministry and sometimes a special church, but the blind, by and large, can worship quite well with the sighted members of the congregation, and so nothing special has to be offered them except counseling, materials and things of that kind, and the pastor can do much in that area.

Pastor Storm suggested that I addresss the Michigan District Convention to keep the needs of blind people before it. When the time for the 1974 convention rolled around, I wrote to President Richard Schlecht, with whom I had served on the Board of Directors for quite a number of years and who was a schoolmate of my wife's, and asked him for a few minutes on the program. This he gladly granted me. In the latter part of June, I arrived at the convention and had my little five-minute slot just after a very difficult vote had been taken on a very controversial question. I told the convention that I was perhaps the most at ease person in the assembly, because I was the only one who was not able to look around and see who was voting for what, so I could not be mad at anybody. This got sort of a chuckle from the audience, and I was on my way. I spoke briefly of the things that the Synod was doing, emphasized that individual pastors can do a great deal, and went right into my climax, which reminded the brethren that handicapped people are particularly the blessed of God. This was my own experience, that God's strength is made perfect in weakness.

My appearance at the convention had some immediate repercussions. Fall is the time for mission Sundays in the Lutheran church, and pastors of congregations look about for a special speaker. Since I was one of a very few blind pastors in The Lutheran Church—Missouri Synod, I found myself with a full schedule for the month of October. I had been called upon to preach at the pastoral conference for our area, the Saginaw Valley Conference, that year, which was a little bit of a tribute, and now I had three Sundays and a Wednesday in which I was to address congregations and, in one case, a student body in a midweek service.

Chapter 8
New Offensives

Now came a period of trial and testing. St. John's, by its tremendous loving support in every way, had shown me that a blind person could serve usefully in a Christian congregation. Now, could the time spent at the Center and the acquisition of some new tools, outlooks, and experience combine with the support of the congregation to enable me to continue a really adequate ministry? The prospect of ever being able to see again was now something of which I never thought. The Lord had given me a feeling of confidence that I would be able to serve Him at St. John's, but I was anxious to move ahead and find some visible proof that this was actually the case.

For quite some time various committees of the church had considered the possibility of starting a daughter congregation. This had been at my instigation, chiefly because I felt that St. John's, with its sixteen hundred communicants, was too large in the sense that we were not keeping our people busy. People were members of the church but were not actively engaged in its program and in the work of the Lord specifically. There were some twenty-three hundred souls, and I was not adequately caring for all of them. A wise plan seemed to be to divide the congregation, take a certain group in some area of town, and start a new congregation, guiding it to a point where it could be self-sustaining. We considered a rural area north of town and even went so far as to make an offer for some property in a very good location near a new high school that was under construction. But we dropped that project when another congregation, Our Savior

Lutheran Church, suffered a split and its pastor left with a sizeable number of people. We did not want to hurt the prospects of the injured congregation in maintaining itself and continuing its ministry by planting a new congregation too near it.

Finally, the general consensus was that we should go to the south of Midland, across the river in an area called Bullock Creek. This was also rural, but it was well built up, and over one hundred and fifty of our members lived in the vicinity. The district mission board was consulted and assured us that they were very much interested in the project but did not have the funds at the time to send a missionary. However, they would be able to take it up after we had made it a going thing. The congregation had $10,000 reserved for this project and was willing to turn this over to a newly established congregation whenever the time seemed opportune.

We had learned something in connection with the Bethel Bible series, and that was that when a group of lay people had been trained to carry out a certain project, they were able to carry it out even if the minister who had initiated it was not there to ride herd on them. So we knew that with some guidance, the lay people who wanted to found a daughter congregation would be able to carry through their project. A survey was held, and it was found that approximately a hundred and forty-some communicant members wanted to take part. And so we began under the guidance of the Mission Board, but chiefly dependent on our own resources. Pastor Brown, as the circuit counselor, held some of the official meetings of the congregation and helped them choose temporary officers and a name for the congregation. I busied myself as much as possible in making contacts, in finding new people that might be interested in a church in that area.

In the meantime, I was placed under a temporary restraining order by my ophthalmologist, Dr. Mesaros. The glaucoma, which had developed in my right eye and caused me considerable trouble at the Center, now came out in full force and could not be controlled by any of the usual means. One day the doctor said it would be necessary for me to go into the hospital and let him operate on the eye. The operation would reduce the size of the gland that secretes fluid for the eye, thus cutting down on the pressure. In due time this operation was performed. I was not confined to the hospital for more than four or five days, but when I came home, I had to be very careful. I was restricted, of course, in the usual lifting, carrying, overexertion, and I was advised that I should not overwork while fulfilling my ministerial responsibilities.

This did hold me back for a while, but I was still keen on carrying out the project of a new congregation. All of my life I had hoped to have a part in such a mission project, and this would be particularly gratifying to me, because I had never been able to accomplish it as a sighted person. Working in the Bullock Creek area as a blind person and reaching out to people whom I had not known before would be a new test of whether a blind person could really offer people the Gospel and effectively bring them into communion with other Christians. So I worked with zeal and prayer and hoped with all my heart that our project would be successful.

God blessed all the efforts of the people who were working to make our new Messiah Lutheran Church not merely a name but a working congregation. Together with some of the lay members, I went about looking for an adequate building in which to hold services. We looked until we finally found a Grange Hall that was well located in the center of the area which we hoped to serve and were told that we could get this building on Sunday mornings beginning in the fall. We would be able to hold Sunday school classes there before or after the church services. The services at the new church had to be dovetailed into those at St. John's, because I would have to preach the early service at St. John's, conduct a service at Messiah, and then go back in time to preach the sermon for the 11 o'clock service at St. John's. A piano was found, and negotiations were also begun to purchase a piece of property so that from the very beginning people would know the church was in the community to stay. A fine piece of property was duly purchased with the assistance of the Church Extension Fund of the district.

The first Sunday in October witnessed the first service at the new mission, and the building was filled to capacity. I preached the first sermon and rejoiced with the members that everybody had turned out. Sunday school began almost immediately, visitors came to the services, and I was in business as far as having calls to make. It was my responsibility to follow up all of these prospects, and I finally came to the point where I was devoting one afternoon a week to this matter. Perhaps to an extent I neglected my work at St. John's, but I felt that it was time well spent. In due time the situation was such that a pastor could be called, and after about a year our direct services— Pastor Brown's and mine—to the new congregation ended.

There was no time to rest on laurels, though. For a long time I had been dissatisfied with our capacity for greeting all the new people that came to Midland. A new nuclear plant was being constructed, some 1,600 people had come into town, and I felt that we had done a very poor job of meeting them. We were not organized to do it well, and although we greeted people at the services, had a guest register and things of that kind, we were missing a great many people as I found out from time to time. I was also concerned about the great many people whom the church never does reach, the people on welfare, unemployment compensation, or relief, the people who live in dingy apartment houses in the poorer residential sections of town or in individual trailers in remote parts of the countryside. All of these people were being missed by the church, and particularly by St. John's, so I was looking for ways and means to reach out to them. My experience at the Center had given me compassion for people who are handicapped by inadequate incomes, education, psychological background, and spiritual background even as they are handicapped by blindness or any injury.

First I asked Pastor Brown, who had been in charge of evangelism for some years, if he would like to rearrange our duties a little and let me have a try at the evangelism program. At the same time, a fund had been established which we called simply "Social Ministry Fund." It was a small fund of a few hundred dollars, but it was to be used to help people in time of need. This could mean any situation at all that brought people into a crisis. I determined that I would make use of some of our lay people, who had already jumped the gun by taking part in an evangelism program at Messiah. At the same time, the chairman of the evangelism program, Del Moeller, and I would take a special course at Utica, Michigan, in August and prepare ourselves so that at the beginning of September St. John's could go into the so-called "Kennedy Evangelism Program" with full vigor.

While I worked on these things, something happened that gave me great personal satisfaction and again reassured me that as a blind person I had not lost standing with friends and associates that I had known for forty years. In June the class of '34 of Concordia Junior College, Fort Wayne, Indiana, held its fortieth anniversary and invited me to speak. Clara and I drove down to Fort Wayne and immediately began to meet people. I was amazed that I could pick up the voices of people whom I hadn't seen for forty years. We had a wonderful time getting reacquainted and reminiscing, and the whole affair was quite a salutary interlude for me.

These days, when I got to the church in the morning at 7:30, the first thing I did was get out my cane and walk around the church a time or two. This kept me in better physical condition and also enabled me to keep up with my cane technique. On some mornings when I had a little more time I would wander around the neighborhood. I would cross several streets and practice making street crossings and going down new streets, keeping always in mind where I was so that I would not get lost. Since there were many people from the church who lived around there, they were forever popping out of their houses and saying, "Pastor, are you lost? Shall I help you get back to the church?"

They did not have the confidence in the cane technique that I had. At other times, people would be driving down the street and would stop and say, "Pastor, can I help you? Are you lost? Can I take you somewhere?"

And I would say, "No. I'm just taking a walk." Then I would explain to them that I was perfectly capable of getting back to the church all right. They would express their doubts, but would let me go. Sometimes if I were trying to cross a very busy thoroughfare, they would stop and say, "Pastor, don't try to cross here. There's too much traffic." It was rather amusing sometimes.

A new test of my mobility and independence came soon after. My mother was in the Lutheran Home in Fort Wayne, somewhat over two hundred miles away from Midland. None of the children lived in Fort Wayne any more, and Mother was quite isolated and dependent upon my visits, so I determined that I would get down there and that I would take a bus. The idea both intrigued me and made me feel uneasy. I had never done any bus traveling on my own, but I knew some of the principles of it. I found out that I could get a bus from Lansing that would take me over to Battle Creek and a transfer there to Fort Wayne would get me in rather early. To go by way of Detroit meant an all-day trip and a late arrival. My drivers were ready again, and drove me down to Lansing. There I got my ticket. My drivers saw me safely aboard the bus, and then I was on my own. It was a kind of uneasy feeling. We had had some talk at the Center about experiences that the blind people had had, and I knew that there are bus terminals and there are bus terminals. Some are new and well staffed. Some are old, in poor areas of the city, and sometimes a hangout for the baser element of society. I knew the bus terminal in Fort Wayne, having picked people up there back in the days of my sightedness, but I knew nothing about Battle Creek.

When the bus arrived at Battle Creek, the driver—and I must say that all bus drivers are very courteous to blind people and helpful to them—saw me into the bus station, found me a seat and told me that my bus would be coming through in about an hour and a half. I sat there and waited patiently. I then remembered that I had memorized the telephone number of a pastor whom I knew in Battle Creek, so I inquired about a telephone, found it, and made a call. I was fortunate enough to find him at home and engaged him in conversation for quite some time. Then I found my seat again, and after a while was approached by a young woman who asked me if I would like something to drink. I said that this would be fine and that I would give her some money.

"No," she said. She would be happy to get me something, and she did. Then she sat down with me and engaged me in conversation. We found out that we were both headed for Fort Wayne and that she was getting off there. So I was going to have no difficulty getting on the bus or getting off, and I was very pleased about this. My worries about a difficult journey turned out to be unnecessary. My friend got me aboard the bus, found a seat for both of us, talked with me, and it was a pleasant trip to Fort Wayne.

There my Fort Wayne driver, Mrs. Melcher, was waiting for me, scooped me up, went out to lunch with me, and took me over to the Lutheran Home where we visited with Mother for a while and agreed to take her out for supper that evening. I spent the night with my cousin, Ruth Horst, and her husband, Mark, and the next morning Mark took me down to the bus station to catch the bus for Detroit. I got aboard in good time with Mark's help and was happy to know that I wouldn't have to make any changes until I got to Detroit.

I was overwhelmed when I got off the bus at Detroit and sensed the largeness of the room into which I was brought, but the bus driver found me a seat, and I sat there for a while and took stock of the situation before I decided that I wanted to be reassured about my bus' time of departure and the location of the gate. I made my way over to the counter which was pointed out to me, and when some kindly person in the line found out that I just wanted information, he shifted me over to another line and told me to follow a rope that was strung there.

I got my information, thanked the man, and asked if he could give me directions to the lavatory. He replied that it was way down at the other end of the building. He called to a young man who was standing there and said, "Soldier, why don't you take this blind person down to the lavatory?"

The fellow said, "Okay," and very kindly let me take him by the arm. The lavatory was kind of an awesome thing. I had no idea how many toilets there were, but there was continual noise, the flushing of toilets, the running of water, people hollering at each other, and odd and sometimes somewhat sinister noises. The young man said, "I'll wait for you here. You go ahead."

So I went ahead. In a few minutes I spoke up, and he said, "Here I am," and took me out into the main seating area and found a seat for me. I asked him if he could look up on the schedule and see anything about the bus. He seemed kind of confused, said he couldn't read the schedule, and didn't see where the gates were numbered. Finally I said, "Don't bother. I've got a lot of time yet." And he went on his way.

So far everything had gone well and I sat down to await developments. The next was that a young lady came forward, sat down next to me and said, "Can I get you something to eat or to drink?"

I hesitated about getting something to drink because I did not like to be pressed into need for a lavatory while I was on the bus. I did not know what facilities they had on buses, whether you had to get off at stations or what the situation was, but finally I accepted the offer of a drink, and she went and got me one. I gave her money and this time it was accepted, and she bought drinks for both of us. She was a congenial young lady and began a conversation, which was interrupted by the young soldier. He stood before me, and I could sense a certain truculence in his attitude. I did not know what the matter might be, but his question was, "Do you have a ticket to Bay City?"

"Yes. I have a ticket to Bay City. That's where I'm headed."

"Well, I want you to look and see if you've got a ticket for Kentucky there too."

I said, "I'm sure I have no ticket for Kentucky."

"Well, I had a ticket to Kentucky until I took you up to the lavatory. Now my ticket is gone. Are you sure that you don't have it?"

This was the kind of thing that I did not like to face as a blind person alone, so I was happy to have the girl sitting behind me—as an interpreter anyway. I told the young man, "Listen, I'm completely blind. If you dropped your ticket, I would never have seen it fall and, if I had, I would never have been able to pick it up."

Well, this stumped him for a moment, but he said, "I'm going to call the police about this matter." And he walked off.

The young girl said, "He's headed for a telephone."

Well, my heart was pure even if my spirit was not as courageous as it might have been in this bus terminal.

The young lady said, "Yes, he's telephoning." Then after a while she said, "He's coming back again."

Next he said, "I've called the police, and told them what's happened. If you've got that ticket, you'd better give it to me right now or it's going to be trouble."

I said, "Young man, you have been very kind to me, but I don't have your ticket. I'm sorry, and if there is any way I could help you, I would like to, but I don't have your ticket."

He said, "Well, you'd better not have my ticket when the police come." And he went away again.

I would not have known what was transpiring except

for the young lady who gave a running report.

She said, "He's over by the information booth again, and he's talking to somebody there. They seem to be arguing." A little later she said, "Here come two policemen." They're coming in the entrance of the bus station. They're going behind the information booth, and they're talking to somebody back there."

After a while they came out, walked over to the young soldier, and talked to him—the girl said quite pleasantly—but then they took him by the arm and said, "Come along with us," apparently, and he quite willingly went along with them. They went out the bus station door, and that's the last we heard or saw of it. We had no idea if he accused me of stealing his bus ticket. I suspected, from his inability to read the signs and from certain other indications that he might have been on some sort of drug and simply confused, that there might never have been any bus ticket or that he might have used it up in some other way. But at any rate, there was no further sign of this young man. I found out that the girl who was sitting next to me was taking the same bus that I was and, with a sigh of relief I relaxed for the first time, because now I could see my way clear all the way to Bay City.

When I came to Bay City, the driver was again very punctilious in taking care of me. He brought me into the bus station, which he said was brand new, and seated me in the first seat of what I presumed was a row. Then I waited for Clara. Ten or fifteen minutes passed and I became a little uneasy, so I went to the ticket office and asked if there was a bus going to Midland yet that night. The ticket agent said that the next bus would be early the next morning. He added that the bus station closed after the last bus came in that evening and would be closed until early the next morning. I said that this might become a bridge that I would have to cross. I had barely gotten seated again when up came Clara and asked, "Where have you been all this time?"

"I have been sitting right here."

She said, "I've been sitting at the other end of this row of seats and reading the paper. I didn't notice when the bus came in or when you came in."

I said, "Well, it's been about twenty minutes."

She said, "Oh, my!" But no damage was done, and off we went to Midland. Thus ended my first expedition by bus alone. It was a little exciting, a little exhilarating, not too commonplace, and I had a feeling that I had accomplished one more thing that a blind person ought to accomplish if he has any sense of independence.

Perhaps two months later I decided it was time for another bus trip to Fort Wayne. This time on the return trip through Detroit, I was directed to Traveler's Aid. The lady asked me what I wanted and I said, "Well, I just wanted to wait until the bus came. I wanted to be sure I knew where the bus left from, and I also wanted an opportunity to go to the rest room."

She seemed a little bit surprised that this was all and said they could arrange it. I was turned over to a very polite young man, who gave me his arm, assisted me up the steps, took me into the noisy rest room, and said, "I'll wait right here for you. You can put your brief case down here. It will be safe." (I'd always carried a brief case with the tape recorder in it since usually I had to either preach or take care of the liturgy when I arrived home on Friday or Saturday evening, and I could thus prepare myself.)

He was as good as his word, and when I was ready, he led me down the steps again, showed me exactly what gate my bus would be leaving from, and then carefully, without letting me lose my sense of direction, put me in a seat that was at the end of a row. Then he said, "Now you walk straight that way and when you hit the wall, turn a little bit to the right, and you'll be at the proper gate."

I thanked him and he went his way but not before I had asked him if I could give him some sort of remuneration. He said, "Oh, no. This is a service that we volunteers render. We believe that as Christians we have an obligation to help the traveler on his way just as they did in the times of Jesus."

I thanked him again and told him how much I appreciated his help. I had not traveled sufficiently to have had many contacts with Traveler's Aid, but this young volunteer certainly impressed me with his kindness, his politeness, and his general Christian dignity.

One Saturday soon after, I went through an experience which shows how a blind person must always be on his guard. Gardening was one of my hobbies, and I loved it not only for the raising of things but for the exercise and recreation that it gave me. This particular July day, I was working in the garden tying up tomato plants. I had placed out perhaps fifteen sturdy five-foot stakes and was tying the tomato plants to them. At that time, Clara was on a visit to Europe visiting our son who was stationed there. I had assured her that I was well able to take care of myself, and up to this point I had been quite successful. But I had not reckoned with my own carelessness.

As I stooped over to tie up the fonds of the tomato to one of the stakes, I brought my eye down squarely upon the top of the stake with sufficient force to cause me instant pain. I rubbed away at the eye, however, blinked a little, let the tears run, and felt no serious damage had resulted. So I went ahead and finished my work in the garden, and then went into the house and did the things that I had to do for Sunday. I ate supper and spent the evening in no particular discomfort.

I went all through the services and the Bible class the next morning, which took from perhaps 8 o'clock till 12:30, then came home and found that my neighbors, the Metcalfs, were frying steaks for lunch. They invited me to join them and I accepted. A little while later Mrs. Metcalf asked me how I wanted my steak done, and I was unable to answer her because of the pain that suddenly arose in my eye. It was a deep and very sharp pain, and I asked her, since she was a registered nurse, to come over and take a look at things. She did and said there certainly was something unhappy going on in my eye. She asked me what I had done, and when I had told her, she said it would probably be difficult to get hold of a doctor, but she would call one to send out some medicine for pain. The medicine did but little good, and after a rather dreadful night, I went to the doctor the next morning. He took a look at the situation and said, "You have caused a tremendous hemorrhage again in your right eye. I don't think we can control the pain because we can't control the hemorrhage. I'll have to put you in the hospital, and the only thing I can do is cut the nerve to the eye and give you relief from pain in that way. We'll have to see then what develops with the eye."

So again, simply because I was a blind person and a careless blind person, I was back in the hospital, flat on my back and waiting for the doctor's verdict. The pain ceased after the operation, except for some minor discomfort from the incision, and the doctor watched the eye carefully for a couple of days. Then he decided that the eye was going to cease hemorrhaging, and it was only a matter of waiting for it to heal. Since I had no vision in that eye anyway, it didn't make much difference what damage the hemorrhage did, so he permitted me to go home, but I was under strict orders to lie down as much as possible and not to engage in any active work. Pastor Brown had been away at the district convention, but he came back by the weekend so the services were taken care of.

Meanwhile a wonderful thing happened. My daughter, who lived in Wisconsin, somehow or other got word that something had happened to me, and since she was not in school at the moment, she came and stayed with me for a week while I recuperated. This was one of the best chances I had had in years to visit with my daughter. She had been in the Peace Corps for four years and, since I had lost my vision while she was there, I had only had a poor image of her when she returned. But now I became acquainted with her as a young married woman, and we spent hours working with some records that I had, putting Braille labels on them so that I could pick out a record and know something about what was on it. She also took care of the cooking and washing, so I had a real vacation. She stayed until my wife came home from her trip.

Life settled down for a little while until we decided that since I could not do much work anyway, we would go off on our vacation at the usual place, Lake James. There I engaged in the therapeutic measure of going fishing with my cousin Wilfred. On one occasion while we were fishing for bluegills, Wilfred performed the unheard of feat of catching seven fourteen-inch catfish in a row. This earned him the sobriquet of "Catfish Kruse" for a long time thereafter.

Somewhere about the middle of August, Del Moeller and I went down to Trinity Lutheran Church in Utica for our clinic on the Kennedy evangelism program. The pastor in charge had been made aware of the fact that I was blind and opened his house to me and my companion, which made my stay even more pleasant. We followed a very tight schedule, started early in the morning, listened to capable lectures on various phases of the Kennedy program, memorized things, and became acquainted with some of the main parts of the Kennedy program. We were briefed on the two basic questions of the Kennedy approach: "If you were to die tonight, are you sure you would go to heaven?" and "If you were to die and face God, and He would ask you, 'Why should I let you into My heaven?' what would your answer be?"

We sang special types of hymns that went well with the evangelism sessions and discussed prayer, approaches, and the various parts of the book which we would eventually have to read. Most parts of the Kennedy program were covered together with demonstrations and presentations. But since the very essence of the program is that you must "go out" and make calls to put what you have learned into practice, we went out three nights, first with an experienced person, then, on the third night, on our own.

Immediately upon our return to Midland, we got together with the seven men and women who had been trained by Pastor Peter Reetz of our daughter congregation, Messiah. These people were full of enthusiasm. The matter of evangelism had been discussed in our church council and meetings for quite some time. Again and again, it was said that we ought to take more aggressive action, and now the time had come for us to take this aggressive action. The seven trainers and I, who had been designated an eighth trainer because we thought that this would be a good number to work with, began to look about for trainees. With no great difficulty we found some rather enthusiastic people. I had to bestir myself to scrape together all of the prospects, all of the leads, that we could find. I searched the records for people who had been married, for people who had been buried, for people who had signed our guest register. We went through the records of the Boy Scouts for unchurched people. We went through the records of the nursery school and, generally, did everything we could to find every last name that was available.

From the very start God blesed the calls which we made in the first aggressive evangelism approach from St. John's Lutheran Church. The very first night some of our trainers had success in their presentation of the Gospel. People received it and even made a commitment to Jesus Christ. Other people actually heard and saw the presentation of the Gospel for the first time outside of church. Many people were a little bit shaken to realize how insecurely they held the teachings of Scripture, how insecurely they held to the fact of their own sinfulness, their complete forgiveness by Jesus Christ and the absolute certainty of eternal life through Him, and as they grasped this for themselves they became more eager to share it with others. As is always the case in a good evangelism program, the first people to benefit in the effort are the people who go out, and sometimes their spiritual growth is most impressive.

When I had been at Utica, I felt that there was sort of a pause in the pastor's voice when he introduced me as a pastor from Midland who was going to take up the evangelism program although he was blind, and a quiet moment while the audience adjusted to this and decided that probably it would be all right. But the people at Midland had been conditioned to a blind person working in their midst, and no one thought that anything would be more proper than to have their blind pastor be one of the trainers and take the lead in making presentations at the beginning of the program. The Lord had prepared me for this in His own way over years in which He had built up my confidence, and permitted me to accomplish things. I now could say in my heart that I felt I could go ahead and be an evangelist in the Kennedy fashion. In fact, one evening I even suggested that it was an advantage to be blind. I asked the evangelists if they did not have some difficulty talking with people through closed storm doors as the season progressed into winter, and they all agreed that this was a problem. Sometimes people would not let the team of three people in, but would converse with them through the storm door. I said, "A blind person has no problem with that situation, because all he does is walk up to the door, say who he is, and then wave his white cane. Immediately the door opens and a cordial voice says, 'Why you poor old blind man! Come on in.'"

As if my cup were not already filled to overflowing, I saw one more prospect of doing something that I had long longed to do. We had made a beginning of it, and now evangelism might help us to carry it out to a fuller extent. This was the social service ministry. During the course of 1975, we had expended several thousand dollars in giving aid to people who were in distress. We served not only families from the congregation; in fact, we more frequently served people who were not from the congregation. Over the years the blessing of God had rested upon the people of

St. John's and the majority of the congregation belonged to the upper middle class as far as income was concerned. They sent their children to college. They lived in homes that were more than adequate. They oftentimes had properties, lake properties, hunting properties, and others in the north country. They had power boats and snowmobiles and camping equipment. They were equipped to live the good, full life that America offers to people with adequate incomes.

But for me, the ideal had always been that the church must reach out to all the people in a community, though this is not an easy achievement. It is difficult to bring together people in an upper income bracket and people in the lowest income bracket. It is difficult to bring together people of diverse backgrounds and cultures. But a common denominator in the Christian church is always Jesus Christ, and His Spirit is the spirit of fellowship, of harmony, and of unity. He can bring these things to pass. The letters of St. Paul to his congregations show that he had preached the Gospel to everyone—the rich, the poor, the educated, the uneducated, the Greek, the barbarian, the Jew, and the Gentile. I felt this should always be the goal of St. John's. Furthermore, our people who had good incomes were Christian people, and they were moved by the words of Christ to help those in need. The Epistle of James and the words of our Lord in which He says that He is going to speak at the Last Judgment are constant reminders to us of our responsibility toward the general welfare of our fellowmen as well as our specific responsibility to preach the Gospel. Now in evangelism and in our social ministry we had tools to reach out as we had never reached out before. The congregation and individual members provided adequate funds to help people in all sorts of needs.

We helped people go to such groups as Weight Watchers and find some assistance there. We provided money for people who had to have abscessed teeth removed. We found clothing for people. We helped people when they could not pay their gas bill, their light bill, or make some unexpected expenditure. People on welfare, for example, have a very strict budget that is laid down by the Social Service authorities, and if anything out of the way comes up, there is no way for them to meet this emergency. They are continually living from hand to mouth, not by desire, but by necessity, and we found that we could oftentimes be helpful on such occasions.

There is a danger, of course, that we might think that by helping people in their physical needs, they will automatically draw nearer to God. This is not at all true unless we combine with the help that we extend the constant reminder that this help comes from Christian people who are motivated by a faith in Jesus Christ, and that the real solution to a man's problems, if he is on welfare, is that he come to know Jesus Christ as his personal Savior, to learn to pray to Him, and find that this Lord will respond to him in all of his troubles.

At first we were tempted to think that there was little thankfulness or gratitude on the part of the people whom we reached in the social ministry effort. But, little by little, we saw that combining the gift with a message of Jesus Christ did have its impacts. Children were baptized; adults made commitments to Jesus Christ. Now and then these people, as out of place as they felt themselves, came to church and were happy to see that our evangelism committee approached them and welcomed them to the services. The help that we extended sometimes got people over a hump, and God's blessing rested upon them so that people who had been on welfare found employment. People whose lives had been terribly disrupted found peace and a feeling of security because they began to appeal to Jesus Christ not only for the forgiveness of their sins but also for help in their earthly position. When the first adult membership class was assembled at the beginning of 1976, some people from this group were in the class. When I became sick and was hospitalized, people from this group came to the hospital; some of them borrowed cars and some telephoned, not because they wanted something—I could give them nothing in this situation—but because they simply were concerned about me. They had come to know me as more than just another person to whom they could run if they were in need.

In consultations with these people, I found that blindness was an asset. People could come to the office and know that I would not be critical of their clothing. I could cast no critical eye upon what they wore or the way their hair was cut or anything of that kind. They knew that I judged them simply by what they said and their responses to the questions which I gave them. They knew that I would speak to them not only of welfare agencies and social services; they knew I would speak to them about the help of God and His love for them and His willingness to respond to them in their need. So, through evangelism, we were able to reach out to these people. It was not possible for one person to reach them all, but many people working together could do it.

One Sunday, I announced that the following week we would have a door offering for the support of our Social Ministry Fund. I told the congregation a few of the things we were doing with this fund and waited to see what the result would be. A door offering at St. John's will generally bring somewhere between $150 and $200. On this particular Sunday, though, we received $900! This showed me that love for the fellow man was in the hearts of our people who on Sunday morning confessed that they loved Jesus Christ. They wanted not only to say that they were Christians and to belong to a Christian church, but they wanted to engage in the Christian life with all of its ramifications.

As 1975 drew to a close and we as a congregation counted all of our blessings, I returned again and again to the realization that the richest, and, in a sense, the most fruitful years of my ministry had come after I had become a blind man. My ministry had never been so exciting, so full of promise, as it was now.

Chapter 9

Full Circle

From the moment the evangelism program for fall 1975 ended, the leaders in our group had begun to plan together with the evangelism people from Messiah for an evangelism weekend. At the same time St. John's was scheduled to hold its first prayer and praise service, to be led by Pastor Donald Matzat and his group from Howard City. In addition to this, our spring evangelism program would start right after the evangelism weekend. My personal goal was to start the adult membership class, and I also wanted to send out a letter to all of the single people in the congregation to see if we could not weld them into some sort of a group. With a lot of work on everyone's part, everything went close to schedule, and I was delighted with the success of the various programs and the spirit shown by the people.

But ever since January 18, I had been feeling a pain in my right leg, a kind of a nagging pain that I laid to various causes. I had had some sciatica before. It might be arthritis. I had twice stumbled violently against a snow shovel leaning against the wall in the garage; maybe that was it. I had had a brief bout with the flu, which had left me with a pain in my right shoulder; perhaps it had gone down now to the right leg. By the evangelism weekend, it had become so nagging I did not go out with the canvassers.

On Thursday evening I came home tired but exhilarated from a meeting with the adults. I was preparing for bed when Clara said there was blood on the bathroom floor. She is somewhat given to overstatement, and I think she said something about "pools of blood everywhere." Of course, I am not aware of these things unless she tells me, but I remembered that I had trimmed a toe nail and possibly had clipped myself doing so. A blind person should be careful about such things, especially when he is diabetic, because they can be the cause of infections. So I put a Band-Aid over what seemed to be a rough spot at the end of my toe.

On Saturday evening when I was taking a shower, my wife again complained about blood on the bathroom floor, so I inspected the bottom of my feet and found that a flap of callous about the size of a nickel had come loose underneath the right big toe, and underneath that was a rough spot. My wife looked at it and said, "My goodness, there's a regular cavity under there. You'll have to see the doctor."

So Monday I went to see Dr. Ittner. He immediately diagnosed a diabetic ulcer and said that it would take at least three weeks to heal. I would have to soak it four times a day in Epsom salts and should stay off it as much as possible. Unfortunately the directions "stay off it as much as possible" meant to me that I could do my work but nothing extra. So I continued to attend morning classes, kept morning office hours, made some calls in the afternoon, and went to necessary meetings in the evening. Every night Mrs. Metcalf, an RN, came over according to Dr. Ittner's instructions. She clipped away at the ulcer, cleaned out dead tissue, and, in general, tidied up the mess.

After a week, the doctor said that everything was going well; I should continue the treatment for another week and keep off the foot as much as possible. So that week I did a little less. But on Wednesday I felt that I must make some calls on various people, people who were sick, people who had to have private communion, and some people whom I had not seen in the nursing home for some time. I traipsed around the nursing home for about two hours and finally could not make any further movement because of the pain in my leg. I had to ask my driver to take me home, and in the evening I even had to call off a children's class. I managed to get by the rest of the week by keeping off the foot and lying down with it elevated as much as possible, and on Sunday I took my part in the services. But when I again presented myself to Dr. Ittner on Monday, he shook his head and said that it was not progressing any further; in fact, it was regressing, and he directed me to make an appointment with a surgeon at once.

Through Dr. Ittner I got in touch with Dr. Robert Brown, and he agreed to see me on Tuesday afternoon. On Tuesday afternoon, however, Dr. Brown's secretary called and said that Dr. Brown was going to be in surgery till 6 o'clock that evening and would not be able to see me. Could she make an appointment for the following week? I said I thought the matter was too urgent, that it was a diabetic ulcer. She then suggested Thursday, and I said I would consult with Dr. Ittner. Dr. Ittner adamantly insisted that Dr. Brown see me on Tuesday, and he made arrangements for me to go to the emergency room at the hospital to see Dr. Brown.

So I came into the emergency room, had some X-rays and blood samples taken, and waited for Dr. Brown. He was as good as his promise and came in at 6 o'clock together with a man who was assisting him that day, Dr. Townsfield. After he had taken one look at the foot, he said, "I have to operate on this immediately. Clear out this room and isolate it because I don't know what kind of an infection this might be."

In a few minutes he had injected analgesic into the toe and laid it open to make it possible for the infection to drain. He said that Dr. Ittner was 100% right. There would have been no hope of saving the foot if he had not been able to begin his work that very evening.

While Clara took the car around to the regular parking lot, I was wheeled to my room. There Clara and I found out what "isolation" meant. The doctor had no way of knowing what sort of infection I had, feared lest it be a staph or some airborne infection that could spread

through the hospital. Before Clara came into the room—before anybody came into the room, they had to put on a gown, a cap, a mask, and rubber gloves. These had to be taken off before they left the room and discarded.

At 7 o'clock then, a new era in my life began and a new experience as far as being a blind person was concerned. It was difficult for a visitor to breathe and to speak when clad in all the protective array, so when a nurse came in, Clara went on her way, exhausted after the tension of the last hours, and the nurse took over in a kindly and efficient way. About 9 o'clock, I went to sleep or into some sort of condition which was to be with me for about four days. I was to learn what isolation meant in a new way altogether.

Years before, when I had been pastor at Rogers City, I not infrequently got up before sunrise and took a little 4-inch telescope that I had down to the lake front north of town, where it was quiet and uninhabited. There I looked out at the stars and watched for the coming of sunrise. It often appeared to me as if I was absolutely isolated on those occasions. No traffic went by on the highway. The lake was perfectly calm, this being a lea shore, and no boats were visible. Only the stars above and the glimmering of dawn across Lake Huron showed any life at all, but no sound, nothing, disturbed the desolation of those early morning hours. Sometimes as I sat on the quiet shore, I remembered how it is described in Genesis 1, that after creation, the Spirit of God brooded over the waters, and I could imagine that that day must have been something like what I was observing here. I felt the isolation of the wilderness, the sea, and space.

I had experienced another type of isolation as a blind person. Sometimes, attending our church conventions, I would be in a hall where hundreds of people were gathered, many of whom I knew as brethren in the ministry and friends over long periods of time. But because of my blindness, I was isolated from them. I could not go up to somebody and say, "Well, hello, Joe! How are things?"

because I could not identify Joe. Sometimes my brethren were not aware of this and sort of overlooked me in the throng, and then I felt that spirit of isolation.

Now isolation came to me in yet a new way. The members of my congregation shied away when they heard that I was in isolation. Some thought that they could not, under any circumstances, come in to see me. The nurses themselves hesitated to come into my room unless it was absolutely necessary, sometimes leaving a number of little chores pile up so they would not have to take off the garb again and again. During that first night, footsteps went back and forth in the corridor, past my door. I heard voices, but nobody came in to see me. I was not being protected from the world, but the world was being protected from me and from any infection that I carried. It would take four days to make a culture and find out whether the infection was one of which the rest of the hospital had to be afraid, or if this special isolation could be lifted, and four days is a long time to a person who is blind, to a person who cannot read, to a person who is feeling very sick.

Then there was the isolation of pain, which takes one's thoughts and bandies them about. There is the isolation of being in an uncomfortable position, in a bed with one's feet elevated at a considerable angle. There is also the isolation of fever which separates a man from his rational thought and even interferes with his prayers. Something like sleep came to me that night, but it was a constant dipping from one nightmare into another. I went from consciousness into slumber and back into consciousness, never knowing just precisely where I was. The delirium even prevented me from saying my prayers properly. I had an intense headache and could not fix my mind on anything. The prayer that came to me was Psalm 130, "Out of the depths have I cried unto Thee, O Lord. Lord, hear my voice. Let Thine ear be attentive to the voice of my supplications." I could begin the psalm, but I could not finish it. And so it went all the long night.

It was a relief when at 4 o'clock in the morning I was slept out in a sense and did not have to face these nightmares. Now I was going to pray. I remembered Psalm 145, "I will extol Thee, O God, my King, and I will bless Thy name forever and ever. Every day will I bless Thee, and I will praise Thy name forever and ever." But I couldn't even continue with a few verses of this psalm. So I tried to pray for my toe, my health, that the fever would go away, but nothing would come clear in my mind. While I had a button to press, I did not press it; in fact, I didn't even think of the button all night. I kept trying to pray, but it was almost as if I were isolated from God too.

Wednesday finally came, and with it the soaking of my foot in a basin and the appearance of the doctor. He clucked over the toe and said, "It will take some time to see if we're making any progress." Then there were further soakings, bandagings, and the meals—a difficult matter because with my feet raised at such an elevation, it was hard to bring my body to a position which enabled me to eat. Food had little meaning anyway. The day passed slowly, and I was almost grateful for the soakings which took up the time. But there was the night to come and with it the fear. Clara came, and I asked her to bring me my tape recorder and some tapes. It had occurred to me that I could carry out a project I had begun at home when I had to spend quite a bit of time with my leg elevated. That was to set down experiences that I had had as a blind person. It was clear that I was going to be at the hospital for some time, and I'd always wanted to do this. Now from 4 o'clock till 8 o'clock in the morning, nothing happened, and as my mind began to clear and the fever went down, I had some little ambition and energy to work on this project.

The second night was very much like the first, but there were not quite so many hallucinations, and my delirium was not quite so deep. The pain in my head was relieved with some kind of a pill, but all during the night I had fantasies about my leg—it was here, it was there, it was here again. In the morning when I woke up and could feel that the leg was just in one place instead of a dozen, and that there was only a slight pain, not pains all over, it was with a feeling of relief.

The second day was much like the first and the third night was much improved. Once I woke, and the thought came to me that my life had come "full circle." Six and a half years before I had been stricken with blindness, and at that time I passed through much spiritual turmoil because I didn't know what was going to happen to me. Was I going to be able to continue my work? Was God keeping me in mind? Did He have a plan for me? Would I regain my sight? All of these things had been on my mind, and I had been confused, worried, and concerned. I had turned to God in prayer, but had no certainty of the outcome. Now I lay in the hospital in isolation after an emergency operation. I was in pain and the doctor had said, "We will be very fortunate if we can save the foot!" These are shocking words to anyone whether he is Christian or not, but they did not have the same impact on me as had the words six and a half years before: "You may lose your sight!" I had become acquainted with the loving kindness of God over those years in a very personal way, and the blessings which God had given me through the congregation, through His own blessing and encouragement, through strengthening my faith, through guiding me from one point to another, could not be forgotten.

If I learned anything through those years, it was that God hears and answers prayer—not always in the way we want it answered, but always in a wonderful way. I had not received my sight, but I had received 150 pairs of eyes. I had lost my vision, but I had gained in my ministry. Never before had I been able to accomplish things as I had after I had become blind, and now though I was isolated in a hospital, the work was going on. However doleful the words, "You may lose your foot," sounded, I could conceive now that the Lord had some answer ready for my problem, and that in due time I would see it. I had always been impatient to get back to work. And I was impatient now, but not nearly as impatient as I would have been before. Blindness had taught me patience.

I could stop worrying about that foot. God would take care of it! And I could go on writing a book about my experiences that would, first of all, review for me once more the wonderful things God had done for me and might possibly help some person—maybe a blind person, maybe simply an afflicted person—to find his or her way through difficulty simply by trusting in Jesus Christ. Jesus' love for man is incomprehensible. When we were yet enemies, Christ died for us; He loves us with a love that never ceases; He blesses us in ways that we cannot know until His kindness is showered upon us.

Chapter 10
Epilog

Dr. Brown had said that I would be fortunate if he could save my foot. And so hundreds upon hundreds of people prayed at St. John's, in our sister congregations, in our daughter congregation, in evangelism groups, prayer circles, prayer chains. My family prayed and my friends prayed. Then one day the doctor said, "I think the foot is safe. Now it is going to be a question of trying to save the big toe."

I said, "Doctor, that's a historic toe, and you must do everything you can to save it."

He said, "What do you mean, a historic toe?"

I said, "Well, if you follow football, you know that all points after touchdown nowadays are kicked by place kicking: one man holds the ball and another man kicks it."

He said, "Yes. I know that."

"Well," I said, "back in 1933, my college, Concordia Junior College at Fort Wayne, Indiana, was playing Howe Military Academy and we were behind 6-0. But then we scored a touchdown and the score was tied. The quarterback said to me, 'Butch, you drop-kick the point!' I had done a lot of practicing along this line, and so I stepped up. The play was called. I drop-kicked, and we won the game 7-6. Now I just wonder if that might not be the last point after touchdown that was drop-kicked in any sort of organized football, and I'm sure that a point after touchdown has not been drop-kicked in professional football for a long time. So do all you can to save that historic toe."

The doctor laughed and went on his rounds.

In a special effort to save the big toe, he sent me to therapy twice a day, and I set some kind of precedent by singing in the whirlpool. Apparently nobody ever did that. On Ash Wednesday I sang every Lenten song I knew. One day I dedicated the morning session to singing German songs, the afternoon to singing Latin songs. One of the girls came over and asked me just what kind of singing I was doing that day. So I explained to her and promised that the next day I would get back to English.

I prayed very earnestly for my big toe. I was almost familiar with God, and assured Him that He didn't need that big toe, but I did need it. The doctor had set a certain Wednesday as the day of decision, and the three days before that, the doctors who examined me said, "The toe looks good. The toe looks good." And even on the day of decision, Dr. Brown said, "It looks good." But then he began to examine it more closely and said, "I'll have to take that back. It looks good here, but it looks bad there. We can't save that toe. The best we could ever hope would be that it would heal partially with an open sore on it. It would be a source of infection and might some day cause you to lose that foot after all."

I had no quarrel with his decision. I trusted him to do what was best for me. A couple of days later, after more sessions in the whirlpool, we went into surgery and I lost the big toe. Whether it ever was sent to the football Hall of Fame in Canton, Ohio, as a historic toe I did not investigate.

I was busy learning something about prayer again. One must always be very humble when one prays to God. We think we know what's best for us. I thought I *had* to have that big toe, but God is so much smarter than I am, that He didn't give me a wish which was a foolish one. He knew what a hazard that toe would be to me if it remained. The doctor understood it, too, and so God let him take off that toe and remove a source of future danger.

Three days after the amputation I could start to try to walk with a walker. The first attempt was a disaster. Four weeks of being flat on my back had left me weak. I struggled from the bed to the door and back again, and that was all, but each day it got easier and I went farther. One day as I was walking down the hall with the walker and the aid of a nurse, I suddenly picked up the walker and walked all the way down to the next ward carrying it. After that I just let it in my room.

The Lord kept me in training for the ministry too. On the same floor with me were a couple of members from the church, and I had a chance to speak with them and become better acquainted with them now than ever before, because we now had something in common—we were all in the hospital. I found four other people who were looking for a church and would be prospects for our evangelism group. I spoke to them about Jesus Christ, and I looked toward the future and working with them.

Dr. Brown was a very taciturn man, and it was vain to ask him for a prediction as to when I could go home. One day I did, though, and he said, "No prediction."

This was March and I said, "Well, June, July?"

He laughed and said, "Before June." Then he made as wild a prediction as he ever did, "Maybe next week."

I was encouraged. I was walking on the foot that had lost its big toe and not having any unexpected pain or discomfort. In fact, it was in connection with stepping on that foot for the first time that I learned a great spiritual lesson. All the time that I had been in delirium, I reached out to God, but really all I felt was pain and confusion. God seemed to be far away from me. In the long night watches I prayed to Him, but I was not aware of any response. It was almost as if I were speaking to Him, but He was being very cool toward me. I knew this wasn't true. I still trusted in God, but something was lacking. All I could really hear was His chiding me—with pain, discomfort, delirium, isolation, separation, and so many other things—until the first day that the doctor said, "All right now. Step down on that foot."

I stepped down on the foot, and for the first time in forty

days there was no pain, and then the Lord got to me. Tears came to my eyes because I recognized His loving kindness and the tender mercy of our Lord Jesus Christ toward the children of men, and especially toward me! It isn't the threats of the Lord that bring us to our knees as much as it is His love that brings us into His embrace.

On the tenth day the doctor came into my room, and I said, "I hope you come as the Great Emancipator?"

He laughed and said, "The only resemblance between me and Abraham Lincoln is that we both have beards, or didn't you know I had a beard?"

I said, "Yes. My wife apprised me of that important fact."

He looked at the toe, and he said, "Wonderful. Goodbye."

And I had to slow him down to ask a few questions about what I should do for the foot, and what I should wear. He told me to come back in five days and he would have another look at it.

Monday noon I came home from the hospital. One of the members supplied transportation because Clara was teaching, and that very evening I was at the elders' meeting. The next day a reader picked me up and took me to the church. I sat down with Pastor Brown to discuss things that would be taking place in the next couple of weeks, the preaching schedule, the hospital work, the nursing homes, and the like. Tuesday evening I was back with the evangelism group. Wednesday morning I sat down with my reader and went through a list of names of people to be visited. Wednesday night I attended church for the first time in six weeks and sat with Clara. At the services she made arrangements with a driver to take me to the hospital the next day where I would make calls for a change instead of being called upon. The following Sunday I was in the pulpit. By the grace of God I was at work again!